More Than a
MOUTHFUL

Published by CelebrityPress™, Orlando, FL
A division of The Celebrity Branding Agency®

Celebrity Branding® is a registered trademark
Printed in the United States of America.

ISBN: 9780983340454
LCCN: 2011930492

This publication is designed to provide accurate and authoritative information with regard to the subject matter covered. It is sold with the understanding that the publisher is not engaged in rendering legal, accounting, or other professional advice. If legal advice or other expert assistance is required, the services of a competent professional should be sought. The opinions expressed by the authors in this book are not endorsed by CelebrityPress™ and are the sole responsibility of the author rendering the opinion.

Most CelebrityPress™ titles are available at special quantity discounts for bulk purchases for sales promotions, premiums, fundraising, and educational use. Special versions or book excerpts can also be created to fit specific needs.

For more information, please write:

CelebrityPress™,
520 N. Orlando Ave, #2,
Winter Park, FL 32789

or call 1.877.261.4930

Visit us online at www.**CelebrityPressPublishing**.com

More Than a
MOUTHFUL

**America's Leading Dentists Reveal How
to Get Healthy and Stay Healthy
by Taking Care of Your Teeth!**

TABLE OF CONTENTS:

FOREWORD

We live in a reactionary world.

When an earthquake damages livelihood, we send aid. ... Building codes are upgraded, inspection rates increase, and committees are formed. When flood waters sweep away progress, we build levies, dams, and barriers in hopes that they won't decimate again. *Humans have never liked pain.* Psychologically, avoidance of pain drives many of our daily decisions and shapes all aspects of life.

Strangely, it is the rare visionary who prepares against future consequence by consuming that ounce of prevention.

Almost all modern medicine is driven by response to symptoms or pain. Nutrition and counseling have found a small niche, but largely, medicine is usually administered after pain or discomfort is discovered.

Dentistry is different. We dentists have always lived in the gray world between prevention and reaction. On the one hand, we have always been there to relieve the exquisite pain induced by a toothache. On the other, we have all dedicated our lives to preventing the pain that fuels our industrial economy.

Dentists spend a major portion of each clinical day trying to convince patients to do things that would keep them away from expensive dental procedures if applied. That is one professional quality that should never be overlooked.

Inside this book you will find a collection of unique professionals. Each one is a true professional and each has a unique flavor that they bring to this proud profession. Many I count as both colleagues and friends.

It is my hope that this book removes a little of the mystery from the world of dentistry, and encourages you to visit your local dentist.

...Maybe you could even visit one before it hurts.

Chris Griffin, DDS

CHAPTER 1

HAVE YOU EVER HEARD A TORNADO?

BY CHRIS GRIFFIN, DDS

H ave you ever heard a tornado? I live in Mississippi so I am no stranger to big storms. We are in a unique area of the country called "Dixie Alley," where weather produces tornados at a clip just barely behind the rate in the Midwestern United States. Before 2008, I had witnessed large hail, fierce winds, non-stop lightning and all the fears that come from tornado warnings, but until then I hadn't actually heard a tornado.

Let me back up for a moment. I have always been the kind of student who attacked my studies and tried to be the best of the best. Everyone needs some area of their life where they feel they are successful and mine has always been academics. When my roommates in college were hitting 'snooze' on their alarm clocks, I was always the one rolling out of bed and shuffling to class so I could keep up my grade point average.

That led to dental school and more academics. I started seeing patients at age 24, and by age 25 I had decided I wanted to be the best dentist in the country. I realize now that there is no such thing, but at that age you can blindly believe in yourself to the point that you head off down a certain path regardless of the obstacles. While I was trying to figure out how to be the best dentist, I came in contact with several great speakers who were proponents of a new thing called "cosmetic dentistry." They had beautiful photos of the dentistry they had done. They had amazing stories of how they had changed people's lives with their magical dental powers. In my mind I had found the Holy Grail of dentistry, so I headed off to be the best cosmetic dentist in the country.

I attended not one, but two very expensive institutes of cosmetic dentistry. I took so many extra educational classes in cosmetics over the next couple of years that by the age of 29, I had qualified for a fellowship in the Academy of General Dentistry. To get that award you have to take 500 hours of continuing dental education and pass a test. Almost no one gets to that point before age 30 and I had done it by taking classes almost entirely devoted to making beautiful smiles.

When all was said and done, I tried to bring my skills to the good people of North Mississippi. For several years I tried to evolve my practice from the kind of place where families came to get cleanings and fillings, to the kind of place where people came to get smile makeovers. A brief definition of a smile makeover would be a combination of several different dental procedures like gum surgery, orthodontics, and porcelain tooth restorations – where a smile looks whiter and more beautiful once finished.

While I loved doing these big cases, I found that they just weren't as fulfilling as I had hoped. Sure, it was fun to make someone's smile better and to improve their self-image. I suppose it also felt good to know that I could deliver services that lots of dentists hadn't learned to do yet. Still, something deep inside kept suggesting that maybe I had spent too much time focusing on these highly-detailed cosmetic cases and too little time on things that I considered "general."

I fought this battle inside myself between being a cosmetic dentist and a family dentist for years. It seemed I could never clear out all of the clutter inside my head to decide which direction I wanted to take my practice.

Nothing quite cuts through the clutter like the sound of a tornado.

It was springtime in Atlanta, and two of my favorite things in the whole world had drawn me there. The Hinman dental meeting is one of the largest in the nation with hundreds of hours worth of classes in just a few days. The Southeastern Conference basketball tournament hosts 30,000 fans with 11 games in 4 days. I love them both and I was right in the middle of it all. In fact, my own alma mater, Mississippi State University, was playing Alabama in the night-cap. Mississippi State was having a good season, but really needed to win that game to guarantee placement into the NCAA tournament that would start the next week.

The game was nip and tuck. The lead changed hands repeatedly over the night and the 30,000 fans inside the cavernous confines of the Georgia Dome never knew that the weather outside had gotten frightful. I was attending the game that night with my father and a dentist friend of mine. As we had made the one mile hike from our hotel to the game, we had remarked that the air was kind of thick. It was hot and humid. But, like I said, we grew up with stormy weather around here and the conditions certainly weren't out of the ordinary for the South in spring. Once inside the air-conditioned Dome, we quickly forgot about the cloudy weather outside and got involved with the ballgame.

As the second half wound down, it appeared that my Bulldogs would advance. They had gotten a little lead on Alabama and, barring a miracle, they would advance to play the next day. Then, lightning struck. No, not literal lightning, but the miraculous happened. A guard for Alabama caught an inbounds pass with just a second left and heaved a desperation 3-pointer toward the goal. It went in. The game was going into overtime.

I was sitting in the Mississippi State section of the crowd and we were all dejected. We should have been walking back to the hotel, and, instead, we were going to have to sweat out another 5 minutes of game time with the distinct possibility that our Bulldogs might lose and miss out on the bigger NCAA tournament. The overtime period began and we were right back to cheering loudly. The crowd cheered loudly.

A couple of minutes into overtime, it seemed to me that the crowd was louder than ever. Then, they got louder and louder. Finally, I told my Dad that this was the loudest I had ever heard any basketball crowd. The decibel level continued to rise. We all looked up and we could see the fabric roof of the Georgia Dome rippling in a way that I didn't think possible. It was becoming obvious that the crowd wasn't making the roaring noise that we were all hearing. It suddenly got so loud that you couldn't even speak to the people sitting next to you without leaning in and shouting in their ear. The players stopped playing and looked up. The giant, hanging scoreboard was now bobbing up and down like a yo-yo. Suddenly, the metal side of the Georgia Dome ripped open like a giant had reached down and jerked the walls apart. Insulation and debris forcefully blew in and the crowds all tried to run for cover.

I had acquired good seats that year down low. We were stuck 35 rows below the safer concrete concourse where people were seeking shelter in the confusion of the situation. There was really no point in my trying to push my way through the mob, because I had finally figured out that we were 'smack dab' in the middle of a tornado, and very soon it would either pass or destroy the building. I decided to just stay in my seat and take my 50 percent chance. Instantly and amazingly the roaring noise stopped, the roof stopped shaking, and things returned to normal. The tornado had passed.

In the aftermath, there was a lot of confusion. The Georgia Dome didn't receive as much damage as it could have, for sure. The officials paused play for about an hour and eventually decided to let the game finish. As we trekked out of the Dome toward our hotel, we saw that the Hinman had received the brunt of the storm. Hotels and businesses right next door had shattered windows and huge chunks missing out of their sides. Large debris was everywhere. The police had closed down the streets and we had to walk a detour to get back to our accommodations. The next day we discovered that the tornado had charged down the street that led from the Georgia Dome to the local hotels that housed both the basketball fans and the Hinman meetings. If that miraculous 3-pointer hadn't gone down and sent the game into overtime, the F3 tornado would have almost assuredly caused a massive loss of life as the fans exited the stadium and walked back to their rooms.

The next day a cancellation of the Hinman and the declaration that the Georgia Dome wasn't fit for play left me with plenty of time for reflection.

Considering that I was a single shot away from possible disaster, was I really doing what I wanted to do with my dental career? I had to look deep inside and come to terms with the fact that I just really wanted to do that "regular" dentistry that I had shunned for the past few years.

Not only did I go home and make that change almost immediately, I developed lots and lots of systems that allowed our practice to make that transition as easy as possible.

One of the biggest changes we made was in the way we presented options to patients. Before the tornado, I had believed that I should only present the kinds of treatments to patients that I would recommend to my own family. Since I would rarely want my own family to get their teeth extracted or get large fillings, I would shy away from recommending them. Lots of my patients may not be ready to do what I would consider ideal treatment right away. I learned to accept that and help them plan accordingly.

I would say that I now encounter the situation where a patient had a painful tooth between 5 to 10 times a day. The patients know that they want to get out of pain, but they don't always understand their options. Let me go through the usual options here that you will encounter when you have a tooth that is painful. We'll assume for the sake of argument that the dentist would find that this pain is caused by an abscess, a common finding in these cases.

1. Root Canal – One way to relieve pain is to do a root canal. This is where the nerve is removed from the tooth and a sealer and filler are placed where the nerve used to be. This reduces the chance of re-infection in the nerve space. If a root canal is performed on a back tooth, a covering called a crown will normally be placed over the tooth to give extra strength.

2. Extraction – The time tested way to get rid of pain is to pull the tooth. There are many reasons to save the tooth, but removing an abscessed tooth will usually get rid of the pain. If you remove a tooth, you will likely want to replace that tooth in the future.

If you decide later on that you want to fill in the space where you removed the tooth, you will have some more options. The 3 most common options are:

1. Partial Denture – This is like a full denture, but not quite so big. It usually has a combination of metal and acrylic and fits against the natural teeth that you still have in your mouth. A partial denture comes in and out and is not permanently secured to your other teeth.

2. Bridge – A bridge is permanently attached to your natural teeth. These are usually made from porcelain and a metal alloy. They allow you to chew very well, but they do require special cleaning techniques to prevent future decay on the natural teeth.

3. Implants – These function as close to natural teeth as possible if you no longer have the original tooth. They are usually made of Titanium and are surgically implanted into your bone. After surgery the dentist usually places a crown over the implant to allow you to chew. These are the best option, but they are also usually the most expensive.

Of course, there are multitudes of variations depending on the specific problems or diagnosis, and some options may not be available to all patients. However, for the patient in pain these are the usual options available.

Nowadays, I have a big, bustling family practice and I couldn't be happier. I still do some cosmetic dentistry, but only for the people who really want it and talk me into doing it for them. That way, they're happier and I'm happier. What I really like is helping people get out of pain in the way that's best for them.

I don't know why it took a tornado to make me realize that.

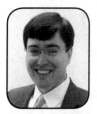

ABOUT CHRIS

Dr. Chris Griffin graduated from the University of Tennessee in 1998 with a DDS degree and began solo practice in Mississippi in 1999. By 2003, he received a Fellowship in the Academy of General Dentistry at the age of 29, and became the youngest person from Mississippi ever to receive the FAGD award at that time. During this pursuit, Dr. Griffin acquired many different general dental skills, including sedation and orthodontics, and brought them to his hometown community of Ripley.

In 2008 Dr. Griffin founded the Capacity Academy to help other dentists learn the most efficient ways to perform dental procedures, focusing on general dentistry. Dentists from all over the United States and Canada have traveled to Ripley to observe and learn his techniques and improve their own patient delivery systems. In Dr. Griffin's opinion, greater efficiency allows the general dentist to produce more dentistry and take more time off. One of his greatest joys in life is spending time with his wife and three children, and he wants all dentists to have the freedom to spend as much time as possible with their families.

Dr. Griffin's many extracurricular activities include the charity, Dentistry With a Heart, coaching and sponsoring multiple little league sports, and serving as an officer in the Mississippi Academy of General Dentistry. In 2010, Dr. Griffin was honored with the Humanitarian of the Year Award by his peers at the Mississippi Dental Association for his community and charitable efforts.

Dr. Griffin still practices solo in Ripley and can be reached at: chrisgriffin@thecapacityacademy.com.

CHAPTER 2

TEETH ARE UP FRONT & PERSONAL – CARE FOR THEM!

BY JANICE FREDERICK, DDS

According to the United States Center for Disease Control, dental caries is the number one disease facing children in the US. Caries is the bacterial infection which causes cavities or tooth decay. Overall dental caries declined in US children from the early 1970s to mid 1990s. A disturbing trend has recently emerged however, and caries in American children is now on the rise.

Primary teeth are the teeth which erupt into the mouth usually between the ages of six months to three years. They are also called deciduous or baby teeth. Although they are eventually lost, it is important to take good care of them.

A child needs teeth to chew and eat healthy foods. A child needs healthy teeth to smile and feel good about themselves. Teeth are involved with speech development. The primary teeth are there to hold the space for the permanent teeth and to help guide them into the proper alignment. Primary teeth or permanent teeth with decay can be sensitive or get infected resulting in a toothache. Children may end up in the dentist's office or emergency room with severe pain and swelling. On rare occasions, children have actually died from lack of proper dental care.

Primary teeth begin to develop *in utero* around weeks 5-6 at a time when a woman may not even know she is pregnant. Women who are pregnant or trying to get pregnant should be sure to have a healthy diet to get the vitamins and minerals necessary to supply the developing fetus. Pregnant moms should take good care of their own teeth and gums. They should keep up with their regular trips to the dentist. Pregnant women may be more prone to pregnancy gingivitis or inflamed gums. Inflammation is not good for the developing fetus – there are studies showing a relationship between gum disease and premature and underweight babies.

When a child is born, little or no bacteria are present in their mouth. Between the ages of six months to two years, bacteria begin to colonize or grow in the mouth. Some bacteria are healthy and some are not. In most cases, the bacteria, which starts to grow in a child's mouth, comes from its primary caregivers, usually Mom and Dad.

The bacteria which forms in our mouths lives in what is known as the biofilm. It is very important for the health of the child that the parents have a healthy mouth. Biofilm and the bacteria living in it can be transferred vertically, for example from a parent to a child. It can also be transferred horizontally. Horizontal transmission would be from siblings or other children that a child is in contact with. Horizontal biofilm transmission occurs also between husband and wife, but that's a subject for another chapter! It is extremely important to create a healthy biofilm in a child's mouth because the biofilm gets harder to control as the permanent teeth come in. Permanent teeth have more grooves and more places for the bacteria to hide. The primary teeth usually start to fall out around age six and the permanent teeth begin to erupt into the mouth. Children with cavities turn frequently turn into adolescents with cavities and finally adults with cavities.

The damage that we see to the primary teeth is usually tooth decay due the infection called dental caries. There are many different bacteria, which can cause tooth decay. The most common are *Streptococcus mutans* and *Lactobacillus*. These bacteria thrive and multiply in an acidic or low ph environment. Do you feel like we are headed back to high school chemistry class?

Enamel on the teeth is the hardest substance in the human body. Enamel's primary mineral is hydroxyapatite which is a crystalline form of calcium phosphate. It is in a constant state of flux. Calcium and phosphate found in the saliva go into the enamel. This is called remineralization. When calcium and phosphate leave the enamel, the process is called demineralization. When you eat, the ph of your saliva goes down. In a healthy mouth, it returns to a neutral ph (ph of 7) in about 20 minutes. If the ph of the saliva is below 5.5, the teeth start to demineralize or decay. The enamel turns chalky white, loses it's luster, breaks down and then the acid gets under the enamel and starts eating away at the inside of the tooth, forming a cavity. If the tooth is not filled, the bacteria will go farther into the tooth and eventually end up inside the nerve. The tooth will then abscess and die. This can be extremely painful and a potentially life-threatening situation.

Plaque is the sticky layer of bacteria and the biofilm that forms on the teeth. It is full of these acid-producing bacteria. Recent studies have shown that even healthy bacteria will start to produce acid if they live in an acidic environment. We need to get this plaque off the teeth and make every effort to keep the mouth free from acid. Sugar is another culprit. It feeds these bacteria, causing them to multiply and causing more acid to be produced.

How can parents have a healthy biofilm to pass onto their children? Parents need to brush and floss their teeth to get rid of the sticky plaque. They need to keep the acidity level in their mouth neutral so that the bacteria in their mouth are not the acid producers. They should see their dentist regularly to get their teeth cleaned and decayed teeth filled.

Plaque will form in a baby's mouth when the teeth start to erupt. Parents may use a clean damp washcloth to wipe the baby's gums 2-3 times a day even before the first tooth erupts. This gets them used to having something in their mouth and makes it easier to incorporate the toothbrush into their care. As the teeth erupt, they too can be wiped off with a clean damp washcloth and even brushed with a tiny toothbrush made especially for infants. The bristle tips may be smeared with just a touch of toothpaste for children less than 2 years old. For the 3-5 year old child, use just a very small pea-sized amount of a fluoridated toothpaste. I recommend that parents plan on brushing (and flossing) their children's teeth until they are 9 or 10. Young children do not have the manual dexterity it takes to brush their own teeth. Never allow your child to run around with a tooth-brush in their mouth. Some children have been injured when they fall and the toothbrush gets propelled into the back of their throat.

Children should not be allowed to suck on bottles of milk or juice for prolonged periods of time, especially when falling asleep. This can lead to baby bottle decay or Early Childhood Caries (ECC). I recommend only water if a child needs to be sucking on something. Juice is very acidic and also has a lot of sugar to feed those acid-producing bacteria. The ph of apple juice is between 2.9 and 3.3! (Remember that teeth demineralize or decay around a ph of 5.5.) A diet high in sugary and starchy foods can drastically increase the chances for decay. Candies that are marketed to kids are often sour (low ph), sugary, and sticky, and can wreak havoc on their teeth.

Pop, soda and sports drinks that are sipped during the day are causing problems in our adolescent population and even in our younger children. Sipping all day is a constant acid attack on the enamel. The saliva has no chance to return to a normal ph to buffer the attack. Both regular and diet soda are acidic. Water has a ph of 7 and no sugar. A popular soda has a ph of 2.4 and a 12-ounce serving contains 10 teaspoons of sugar. It's diet alternative has no sugar, but its ph of 3.1 is still low. The Minnesota Dental Association website has good educational information in their "Power of Sour on Your Teeth" and "Sip All Day Get Decay" campaigns.

When should you bring your child into the dentist for their first exam? The American Academy of Pediatric Dentistry recommends a visit to the dentist when the first tooth erupts. This is the opportunity for the dentist to check out the baby's mouth and also instruct the parents in good oral care for their child. The most frequent recommendation for dental checkups is every six months, however, there are cases where I see higher risk children every three months.

Pediatric dentists are dentists who have completed 2-3 years of extra training just to treat children. Their offices cater to the younger crowd. Many general dentists also see children. As a mom myself, I enjoy seeing children. I was fortunate to grow up with a father who was a dentist and was taught early on the importance of good dental care. Making your child's visits to the dentist a pleasant experience can set them up for a lifetime of good dental health. Most children do extremely well at their dental appointments if their parents present it as a positive experience. Unfortunately, waiting until they have obvious problems can lead to a frustrating experience for the child, the parent and also the dental team.

As the children get a little older, around 2-3 years, most will sit in the chair and allow us to polish their teeth. The hygienist will show Mom and Dad the proper brushing and flossing technique for the child. Over time, calculus (sometimes called tartar) may begin to build up. It is hard and cannot be removed with a toothbrush. The hygienist will also clean this off with special instruments. Older kids will often need more encouragement on good oral hygiene as they become more independent.

Gingivitis is a mild form of gum disease. The hygienist will explain the importance of removing plaque not only to avoid cavities, but also to prevent gingivitis. Gingivitis causes the gums to become red, swollen and bleed easily. If left untreated, it progresses into *periodontitis* – which causes the body's natural immune system to kick in and start to break down the attachment of the gums to the teeth. This leads to bone loss and eventual tooth loss. Refer to chapter 12 for more information on the deleterious effects of periodontal disease on the entire body. Juvenile periodontitis is a rapidly progressing type of gum disease which may first be detected in adolescents ages 11 to 13. It is extremely important to detect and treat it early.

Tobacco use often starts in adolescents. Dental teams will explain to your teen the risks associated with both cigarettes and smokeless tobacco products. These risks include decay, gum disease, nicotine addiction and oral cancer. According to a recent study, the levels of smokeless tobacco use in US males ages 12-17 increased from 3.4% in 2002 to 4.4% in 2007. Another recent survey (2009 Youth Risk Behavior Surveillance) showed that 19.5% of high school students smoked cigarettes during the 30 days before the survey.

Your dentist may recommend fluoride rinses in children who can spit. Fluoride speeds up the absorption of healthy minerals by the enamel and makes it harder, shinier and more resistant to the acid attack. Your dental team may also apply fluoride treatments and varnishes.

Xylitol is also emerging as a bigger player in the care of teeth. A recent study done in Finland showed that a daily dose of 5 grams of xylitol in mint or gum form had a 50% reduction in tooth decay (children 10-12 years old over a two year period) versus the control group. Other studies have shown a reduction in ear infections in children as well. Xylitol is a naturally-occurring sugar. Bacteria cannot break down xylitol into acid as they can with other sugars such as sucrose, fructose and sorbitol. They also take in less other sugars, which decreases acid production. Xylitol also appears to make it more difficult for bacteria and the biofilm to adhere to teeth. Xylitol can be found in gum, mints, rinses, breath sprays and as a granulated sugar substitute.

Dental sealants are another way to prevent cavities in the "hard-to-brush" pits and fissures of the teeth. Most dentists recommend carefully placed sealants on the 6-year or first permanent molar and also on the second or 12-year molar. They may also be placed in the grooves of the more anterior teeth. Sealants can cut the risk of decay, but must be monitored carefully by regular dental visits. Decay can still get underneath them and spread rapidly if not detected

Flossing is a difficult habit to acquire, but it is important. Flossing helps to clean the teeth where the toothbrush cannot reach. Parents will need to floss their children's teeth until they have the manual dexterity to do it. If it becomes a part of the daily routine, you will usually see less tooth decay and also less gum disease.

What other things are dentists watching for in children and adolescents? We are watching the development of the upper and lower jaws. With an appropriately-sized jaw, there is usually room for the permanent teeth. Jaw size can be influenced by the airway. Dentists are concerned about breathing. Breathing through the nose is healthier than breathing through the mouth. Air that goes through the nose is combined with nitric oxide, which is a vasodilator. This means that when this air reaches the lungs, it is easier to get oxygen into the bloodstream. Can you imagine how difficult it is for a young athlete to get adequate oxygen into their body without good breathing? Also, breathing through the mouth causes a dryer mouth. Dryer mouths have less saliva to buffer the acid attack and the risk for decay goes up.

Children who breathe primarily through their mouth will usually have a narrower upper arch and less space for their permanent teeth. Enlarged tonsils and adenoids can contribute to this problem. Allergies which make it difficult to breathe through the nose may need to be treated.

Pacifiers, thumb sucking, finger habits and tongue habits can also affect the growth and development of the jaw. Most children stop sucking on fingers and pacifiers on their own between the ages of 2 and 4. When a child continues this behavior, it can cause the teeth to flare out, causing an open bite. The open bite can affect the tongue position, the developing swallow pattern and also speech.

People respond positively to other people who smile. Self-esteem can take a nosedive in children who do not feel comfortable smiling because of ugly decayed teeth, crowded or protruding teeth. Orthodontics or braces can straighten teeth and make it easier for children to smile naturally. Crooked teeth are also more difficult to clean. This can lead to more decay and an increased risk for periodontal or gum disease as an adult. Some types of crowding problems need to be corrected while the jaws are at a certain stage of development. This is another reason children should be seen by their dentist on a regular basis. Appliances can be placed which widen the jaws, allowing more space for the permanent teeth. These appliances can also open up the airway making it easier to breath through the nose. Missing this window of opportunity can cost more money in the long run and also compromise the final treatment outcome.

Orthodontics has become more streamlined since I had braces. Brackets or braces are bonded to the front teeth rather than cemented with big metal bands. We have many more tricks to move teeth into their appropriate position. There are also clear plastic tray aligner systems which can be used in selected situations to move and align teeth.

Sleep disordered breathing in children is an emerging science. It may be tied in with airway issues. Does your child sleep soundly, or are they restless? Imagine how hard it is to get through the school day when you have not had a good nights sleep. Will you child's grades suffer? Can he or she concentrate at school? How would this affect them socially with their peers? Don't be surprised if you dentist asks about your child's sleep.

Dentists are also watching for signs of wear on teeth. Many children will grind their teeth while they are asleep. Although this is rarely a problem for the baby teeth, it can be a problem when the permanent teeth start to erupt. Tongue piercing can cause chipped teeth. It can also cause bone loss to the lower anterior teeth. This bone loss is usually permanent, and these teeth will require gum grafts to help protect the remaining bone. Another type of wear can be the result of bulimia or acid reflux. Your dentist is often the first health care provider to detect these important and potentially life-threatening medical conditions.

Children who participate in a sport that carries a significant risk of injury should wear a mouth guard to protect their teeth. This includes a wide range of sports like football, hockey, basketball, baseball, skateboarding, gymnastics, and volleyball. Preformed or "boil and bite" guards can be bought in most sport stores. Dentists can make more customized and comfortable guards. Dentists know the tremendous life-long costs associated with broken front teeth. Fractures and trauma can lead to the need for bonded fillings, root canal treatments (if the nerve dies), eventual veneers or crowns. Sometimes teeth are lost all together. Mouth guards can also help protect children from head and neck injuries such as concussions and fractured jaws.

Hopefully, I have convinced you of the importance of good dental habits and regular dental care. Dentists and their teams are focused on prevention of dental problems. We want you and your children to enjoy healthy teeth, gums and a beautiful smile for your entire lifetime.

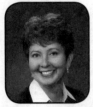

ABOUT JANICE

Dr. Janice Frederick received both her Bachelor of Science degree and Doctor of Dental Surgery degree from the University of Minnesota. She joined her father in his dental practice where they practiced together for over 20 years. Her current office is located in Mendota Heights, Minnesota.

Dr. Frederick is a member of the American Dental Association, the Minnesota Academy of General Dentistry, the American Academy of Cosmetic Dentistry, the American Academy of Dental Sleep Medicine and the Minnesota Academy for Comprehensive Dentistry. She attends over 100 hours of continuing education each year.

Outside of the office, she enjoys gardening and photography. Dr. Frederick has two children and lives in Minneapolis with her husband Dan.

CHAPTER 3

YOU ARE GOING TO DO WHAT TO MY MOUTH?
– UNDERSTANDING DENTAL TREATMENT RECOMMENDATIONS.

BY CHARMEN DOUGLAS, DMD

A common scenario is a patient visiting a local dentist for their regular check-up and cleaning and is horrified by the news that they have GUM DISEASE. The dentist and the hygienist say, "You need treatment right away." Next to the fear of pain from dental treatment, the fear of losing teeth ranks second on the Richter scale in this patient's mind.

It is difficult to understand how a person can be inflicted

with a disease and not see any sign or warning such as pain or bleeding. Visions of torturous procedures race rapidly through the mind of this patient, while the hygienist is explaining the treatment in dental jargon that a master scientist would have trouble understanding.

The fundamental art of communicating to patients in laymen's terms was lost somewhere in the first year of dental school. Dental professionals communicate treatment as if they were giving a lecture at their local college. "We must appear intelligent and sophisticated with our words and mannerisms in order for our patients to believe we are excellent clinicians" are the thoughts of most dentists. The reality is that the patient did not hear a word of what the dentist said, because the technical words were not understood with all the dental terminology. As the patient tries to redeem his senses and nods feverishly to agree, so the hygienist would stop showing horrific pictures of untreated gum disease, the only thought that runs through the patient's mind is the location of the nearest exit. To add insult to injury, the dentist says "the cost of the treatment will be $1,200 if you do not need surgery now." As the blood returns to the patient's face, the patient thinks in his mind, "this must be a bad dream… I just wanted a cleaning." The patient leaves confused and the dentist feels defeated because the patient does not understand the significance of the treatment to prevent the loss of teeth. Where did the communication fail?

Little do we know as dentists, patients do not want a scientific explanation all the time; they want to understand, "How can I possibly have such a terrible disease and not feel pain?" Patients have a value for treatment and service that addresses problems they can see or feel. Patients are not moved by problems they believe are not priorities. For example, if a patient is looking forward to the day he or she can take out their teeth at night and not worry about dental pain, they will not be interested in the benefits of saving teeth with gum treatments, they want dentures. If a patient is not concerned about saving a tooth with a root canal procedure, the dentist's words goes in one ear and out the other as the patient looks at their watch. Patients develop their own value for treatment and services. One person's fear is another person's desired dental solution. An experienced clinician will learn that patients will not get treatment unless they feel there is a need. The few patients who agree to treatment without understanding the benefit of the service will continue to wonder if it is truly necessary. The dentist is often perplexed about why patients do not want to take care of their teeth.

Patients do want to take care of their teeth, that's why they seek maintenance, care and cleanings. However, somewhere down the line somebody said dentistry was going to last forever or if I brush my teeth everyday, three times a day, I will not have any problems. For these folks, the tooth fairy took a sabbatical. Patient 'A' now sits in the dental office with the harsh reality that the teeth Mother Nature gave him are failing him, and he asks, "What do I do now?"

This is where the complications for the dentist begin; they must explain and resolve all the patient's misconceptions about teeth in a matter of 5 minutes, before the patient stops listening. The hygienist will pull out their best models and best graphics to get the point across. "Teeth are important." …"Cavities will destroy your teeth." …"Don't pull your teeth, you will create big spaces." … "Missing teeth can lead to pain in the jaw joint." …"Headaches and jaw pain related to your bite problem stem from the missing teeth." The sounds of explanations ring on and on in the mind of the patient for days. The complex options and alternatives only confuse the patient more, and the patient leaves in a worse mental state than when he walked in. Patient "A" will probably not go through with any recommended treatment. He will suffer silently and return to the dentist when the disease has advanced to a stage where the tooth cannot be saved. If only the dentist was able to communicate at a level of understanding with patient "A".

Patient "B" enters the dental office with hopes of enhancing her smile with a cosmetic enhancement procedure seen on television. Patient "B" has been going to her dentist since she was a young child. She landed a high profile job in the public eye and believes her smile may impede further growth in the company. Patient "B" knows her confidence will go up with a few cosmetic treatments. Patient "B"'s dentist is very conservative and does not understand why she wants to alter her teeth with minimal invasive cosmetic treatment. He thinks her teeth are fine and tries to talk her out of the procedure. Patient "B" leaves the dental office with only the cleaning and exam again. Patient "B" vows to find someone who understands the importance of her dental cosmetic enhancement. Patient "B" researches on-line and finds a dentist who communicates on her level and understands her needs and wants. Patient "B" gets the dream smile she always wanted and never looks back to continue further treatment with her childhood dentist. If only the dentist was able to communicate at the patient's level of interest.

These scenarios occur often when the patient and the dentist do not see eye-to-eye. To the dental professional's dismay, communication of our wealth of knowledge is a challenge. Even though all dentists have graduated from a reputable school, it does not mean the skill of communication was mastered. Dental School prepares dentists for the clinical challenges of treatment, but does not train the dentists appropriately for rejection of treatment. Discovering the dentist's communication style is the most important part of the dental process. The seasoned dentist will know that there are many reasons why a patient may not accept treatment at the discovery appointment. A patient's reluctance to complete a recommended treatment will vary due to cost, fear, time and the lack of understanding of the treatment. The why's, how's and when's of the treatment and its goals must be revealed.

One of the frequent mistakes many clinicians make is to try to impress the patient with sophisticated clinical terms during a discussion. Somewhere we were told that the bigger the word you use, the more professional and knowledgeable you are. The reality of the fact is that the patient thinks you are *scary* and likely does not understand one word you said! Meanwhile, most of the common disorders are non-life threatening. However, the dentist knows untreated dental conditions can, and will, lead to great destruction and overall medical compromises. To the dentist's dismay, this failed communication style turns patients away, and either they do not accept recommendations or they go to another dentist who speaks their language.

There is a solution to this ongoing dilemma. You can learn to appreciate and embrace the passion of your dentist's desire to help you save your teeth and decrease your susceptibility to medical complications. Here is a translation of some of the most common treatments and diseases of the mouth. These are the most common and misleading clinical terms that make patients ready to jump out of the chair:

Periodontal Disease: Better understood as gum disease. This is a condition where the bacteria growth in the mouth reaches levels that initiate your immune system; the body produces a natural defense to protect you from the invasion of bad bacteria. What we see and smell are bleeding gums and/or morning breath. The mouth has more bacteria than any other part of the body. When the levels of bad bacteria outnumber the good bacteria, we get gum disease. Over 75% of the population may experience some form of periodontal disease in their lifetime. Later on in the chapter you will see solutions on how to maintain and prevent periodontal disease (gum disease).

Root Plane & Scaling: This is gum treatment for periodontal disease. I once had a patient who admitted to visions of all the teeth being removed, cleaned and put back in the mouth during gum treatment, while her other dentist tried to convince her to complete gum therapy. Needless to say she was pleasantly surprised and relieved at how easy and painless the treatment really was with the proper numbing and good clinical hands. Gum treatments do not have to hurt. Taking the proper precautions before and after treatment reduces anxiety and discomfort. This treatment can prolong your life by reducing the amount of bad bacteria that circulates throughout the body; at the same time it also helps to support better heart function. Patients with a compromised heart function and high levels of bacteria may require oral medication prior to treatment conjunction with gum treatment.

Root Canal: One would think this was a four-letter word in

dentistry. I am curious to know who started the rumor that "all root canals are bad and painful." Root canal procedure is the treatment to remove painful and infected nerve tissue in the tooth. If you had a severe toothache, trust me, a root canal feels much better. In fact, root canals do not have to hurt. If precautions are taken before during and after the root canal treatment, a patient can resume normal activity without the preoccupation of discomfort. Normal activity is encouraged, and you must remember to take your medication as directed.

Anesthesia: This term may be a little confusing. Some patients think this is the stuff used to put people to sleep. Most often it is referred to as the material used to numb an area in the mouth in order to avoid discomfort. I try not to use the "P" *(pain) word*, because for some people, this word sends cold chills down their spine when mentioned.

Novocain: This is a common word used in the past to describe a numbing technique.

Cavities: Holes in the tooth. It is the overgrowth of bacteria that leads to decay, breaks down the surfaces of the enamel, and forms holes in the tooth. These allow additional bacteria to growth inside the mouth. When the decay is left untreated, it travels the depths of the tooth to invade the nerve. The treatment for cavities is the procedure called "filling". If bacteria are allowed to travel into the nerve space, the nerve or the entire tooth must be removed to eliminate discomfort.

Fillings: The material used to correct the defect of a cavity after the bacteria is removed. Various options of fillings are available such as **amalgam** (silver), **resin** (white medium strength material), and **ceramic** (white hard high-strength material usually used in teeth with little tooth structure after bacteria *decay* removal; it mimics the look and strength of enamel).

Crowns: AKA *Caps*. A cap is a cover to protect and restore function to a tooth that has lost the ability to withstand normal biting forces. Broken teeth, root canal teeth or teeth with large defects will experience greater longevity with a protective cover that surrounds the entire tooth.

Onlays: A protective covering used when a substantial amount of tooth structure is missing, and the likelihood of repeat breakages will occur with a resin filling. Onlays are used when there is still a good amount of tooth structure remaining and the tooth nerve is healthy.

Veneers: Coverings for the front teeth to give an enhanced appearance. Instantaneously, defects, mis-shaped teeth and discolorations disappear. Very natural porcelains or ceramic coverings match the other existing teeth in natural and artificial lighting.

Bridges: We like to think of these as bridging the gap or spaces. It is a means of replacing a missing tooth with a permanent non-removal connection of crowns or caps. It gives the illusion a real tooth is in place. It requires at least two teeth, one in front and one behind the space to anchor the false teeth. Tooth structure removal is needed to make room for the metal and/or ceramic material better known as porcelain ceramic. The result is a natural-looking smile without having to take your teeth out at night.

Implants: A treatment option to replace teeth with a permanent tooth with or without connecting teeth. The tooth is placed into the missing space and the bone grows around the implant tooth as if it was a natural tooth. It resembles and feels like a natural tooth after the crown is made. There are two or more parts to an implant crown. Surgery healing varies between 3-6 months on average, unless new healthy bone is needed prior to implant surgery. This option does not involve tooth structure removal from healthy natural teeth.

Dentures: The teeth you take out at night. May either be a full set of teeth, or a partial set of teeth if some natural or implant teeth remain in the mouth.

Cleaning: This is the most important aspect of dentistry. Professional cleanings are solutions to reduce the dangers of developing large amounts of bacteria, which are harmful to your health, teeth, and gums. It will also save you costly treatment if you maintain your existing dental work with professional cleaning maintenance. Some people develop bacteria rapidly and require more frequent cleaning to maintain gums and teeth. *All in all, cleanings are one of the best investments to prevent costly dental procedures and prevent medical complications associated with bacteria formation in the mouth.*

Overall, with better communication and understanding, patients will not be overwhelmed by treatment recommendations. Steps should be taken by the patient to seek dental providers who communicate in a language they can understand. Not everyone is well versed in dental jargon, so do not feel you are alone in this quest to seek better options to achieve a healthy nice smile. Research your options, and ask for a consultation to develop a rapport with your dentist and hygienist. Find a dentist who will communicate to you your needs, at a clear level of understanding. Don't miss the opportunity to improve your dental and medical health with sincere communication and guidance. Embrace your dental health…maintain your nice smile. You will wash away years from your appearance and feel better in the long run.

Keep smiling!!!!!!!!!

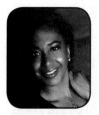

ABOUT CHARMEN

Dr. Charmen Douglas is an Oral Physician Dentist and is currently in private practice within the Southern Jersey Area. Charmen Douglas has a Bachelors of Science Degree in Nutrition and a Doctorate Degree in Dental Medicine. Dr. Douglas is the CEO of Beautiful Smile, LLC and Founder of, Give Back A Life Foundation LLC; which serves to provide up to $30,000 of dental services to domestic violence victims each year. During her 19 years of practice in the field of Dentistry, Dr. Douglas has been appointed to the National Dental Association's House of Delegates, New Era Dental Society's Executive Board, and elected to serve on the Executive Board for the South Jersey Medical Association.

Dr. Douglas has been recognized for her advanced work in medical-dental health, and Beautiful Smile LLC is the first Dental group to receive a Forbes Enterprise Award. Commitment to service in the community is a top priority for Charmen Douglas. She believes in educating the public on alternative treatment options and daily modification of everyday habits, to promote better overall health and stronger teeth. Dr. Douglas has become one of the leaders in medicine and dentistry, through the use of non-invasive therapies such as neuromuscular dentistry, diet modification, and soft tissue management. The public is unaware that some chronic medical conditions are complicated by a disease found in the mouth and/or head and neck.

Dr. Douglas is a member of the Academy of General Dentistry Speaker's Bureau, and lecturers to other dentists about the effects of toxins found in our mouth that can complicate existing cardiac and respiratory conditions. Dr. Douglas continues to participate with New York University as a practice Investigator for the development and modification of our dental procedures – to better serve patient's health and medical needs.

Charmen has been a guest of CN8 News and MDTV as an expert on sleep apnea and cosmetic therapy. South Jersey's Courier Post featured an article on Dr. Douglas as an expert in aliments associated with gums.

Some feedback comments from past interviews are as follows:

"You should get a lot of calls from the interview"

~ Arthur Fennell ~ CN8

"Very informative and interesting"
~ Shawn Rheau ~ Courier Post

Dr. Douglas enjoys tailoring her talks to suit different ages and interest groups. She is very likeable and has become an excellent person to interview, by her captivating her audience with a layman's approach to everyday health issues pertaining to the mouth and the surrounding structures.

CHAPTER 4

THE MYTH OF LONG TEETH & RECESSION

BY GREG PHILLIPS, DDS

When I was a young boy, I was standing in line at the grocery store with my mother when I heard one lady say to the other, "Him? Not a chance. He's far too long in the tooth!" I stood there puzzled. Were they talking about Dracula? I waited until we were loading the groceries into the car before I asked my mother what the lady meant by "long in the tooth." She smiled and gave me that age-old answer, "Ask your father."

She was justified in the hand-off, I guess, because my dad was a dentist, after all. However, he was also a man of few words. When I replayed the conversation to him and asked for an explanation, he closed his newspaper for a second, turned his head, said "That fellow is old," and resumed reading his paper.

Ohhhkaaayyy, I thought. There's a cause-and-effect. The older you get, the longer your teeth get. I furrowed my brow. When exactly do they start growing again? How long do they get when you are really, really old. Will they grow over your lips? How could I find out? Ha! The oldest person I knew was our next door neighbor, Mrs. DiGeorge, a widow with blue hair and a walking cane. I found her in her front yard watering her flowers. I made small talk for a few minutes and then I said, "Will you smile for me, Mrs. DiGeorge?" She looked confused, but did so. Her teeth looked the normal size to me. "Did your teeth used to be smaller?" I asked. She smiled again and turned back to watering her flowers. "No, dear" she said, "but they used to be real."

It was not until I was in dental school that I learned that the natural causal relationship between age and "long teeth" is a myth. A tooth *appears* longer than normal when the gum tissue holding it in place is worn away to reveal more of the tooth. In other words, the tooth is the same size it has always been; it's just a little more naked. The technical name your dentist will use for the disappearance of the gum tissue that held your teeth in place is *recession*.

After more than 30 years in practice, though, I am still amazed by the prevalence of the dental myth. When the loss of tissue around a patient's tooth is pointed out, I will ask him or her if this recession causes concern. The typical response? "Dr. Phillips, I'm just getting old. It's natural." No, no, no! "Long teeth" do not occur as a natural result of aging! This chapter is my attempt to debunk that myth once and for all; it will explain the problems with losing gum tissue, the real causes of gum recession, and the techniques for ensuring healthy gum tissue.

Patients often have difficulty understanding that gum recession is a problem; they frequently comment, "Dr. Phillips, it doesn't hurt; why worry?"

Three main problems generated by recession are:

1. **Loss of teeth:** As gum tissue recedes, the bone and supporting structures of the tooth disappear also. If this erosion becomes so severe that the tooth lacks sufficient support, it will loosen, and ultimately fall out.
2. **Sensitivity:** As many patients have unfortunately discovered, as the gum tissue recedes, more and more of the root surface is exposed. An exposed root surface leads to a painful sensitivity to hot and cold liquids and to sweets.
3. **Cosmetic damage:** When one or more of the front teeth lose gum tissue, the smile can be damaged. In particular, the highly visible canine (or "eye tooth") is one of the most common teeth to suffer from gum loss; unfortunately, once the canines are exposed, they can have a fang-like resemblance.

So, even if gum recession does not immediately hurt, it can pose long-term dangers.

To address the dangers of gum recession, we need to understand the following causes. Every day in my office, I have the opportunity to interview new patients. One of the first questions I ask them is "What kind of toothbrush are you using?" In one week, three of my first four patients stated they used a medium or hard toothbrush. When asked the reason for that choice, one patient could not remember the reason, the second patient believed the harder the toothbrush, the better the cleaning job it would do, and the third said her dentist recommended the choice (a surprisingly frequent reason).

Why do I focus so much on toothbrush selection? In my office, the number one cause of gum recession is **toothbrush abrasion** brought on by patients who use the wrong toothbrush. Medium or hard toothbrushes have stiff bristles that lack the subtlety to gently penetrate and massage the gums into health. Instead, these stiff bristles skate roughly over surfaces and apply so much pressure to your teeth and gums that, over time, these bristles operate like sandpaper: they dig grooves into the enamel of your teeth, and they thin and then ultimately erase the gum tissue. Quite frankly, the only legitimate use for a toothbrush with such stiff bristles is to scrub clean the grout between the bathroom tiles! These toothbrushes should be sold in the hardware section of pharmacies and grocery stores.

Add to the wrong toothbrush an **improper brushing technique**, and the potential for recession becomes severe. What is an improper brushing technique? The worst way to brush your teeth is to concentrate solely on the teeth and to saw at them brusquely in a horizontal fashion. It is a recipe for disaster.

Besides using a stiff toothbrush and brushing improperly, other causes of gum recession include:

- *periodontal disease*: There is a common misconception that recession and gum disease are one and the same. Gum disease, otherwise known as *gingivitis* or *periodontitis*, may indeed cause loss of gum tissue, but gum recession is not necessarily a sign of gum disease.

- *prominent roots of teeth in the dental arch*: When the teeth are crowded inside the dental arch of the mouth, some teeth can push forward over others. This relocation can pull the gums tightly and cause thinning and then erosion.
- *muscle attachments*: Muscle attachments, such as the *frenum*, can pull too tightly upon the gums and lead to recession.
- *excessive bite force on teeth or a single tooth*: The up-down motion of clenching and grinding and the side-to-side motion of *bruxism* are two of the forces that can lead to recession. Another source of excessive force on teeth are the stress caused by a problematic occlusion (the way your teeth fit together); for example, teeth may be crowded or misaligned. When this poor alignment occurs, it causes interference in the bite and leads to too much stress on individual teeth and thus on the gums and supporting structures.

These are certainly significant causes that your dentist can help you address. Here, I aim to go after the cause I see on a daily basis, the cause that has the easiest solution: toothbrush abrasion.

The two steps for preventing toothbrush abrasion are as follows:

1. Use a soft toothbrush.
2. Use the proper toothbrush technique.

Simple, yes? But remember that three out of four patients I interviewed in one week alone were using a medium or hard toothbrush. More incredible to me, according to my patient, there are dentists still recommending the use of these stiff brushes.

The proper toothbrush technique may initially seem complicated, but with practice, you will quickly get the hang of it. My recommendation is the following Modified Bass Brushing Technique because it encourages the thorough but gentle removal of plaque from your teeth:

- **Prepare**: Hold the toothbrush horizontally (sideways) against a small area, two or three teeth, with the bristles touching your gums. Tilt the brush upward at about a 45-degree angle so the bristles aim for your gum line. For the inside of your tooth, you can hold the toothbrush vertically (up-and-down) for ease of use.
- **Dislodge bacteria and plaque from the gums**: Use short strokes to move the head of the brush back and forth, and keep the tips of the bristles in contact with the tooth and gums. The tips of the bristle should stay in one place, and the head of the brush should vibrate back and forth. You want the bristles to slide gently under the gum to dislodge the bacteria that hides in the pockets around the tooth at the gum line. Wiggle the brush about 5 to 10 times per area on both the inside and the outside of the tooth.
- **Remove the plaque**: Roll the brush so that the bristles sweep from under the gum line toward the tip of the tooth. In essence, flick the plaque away from under the gum. Perform on both the inside and the outside of each tooth.
- **Clean the surfaces**: To clean the biting or chewing surfaces of the teeth, hold the brush so the bristles

are straight down on those surfaces. Gently move the brush back and forth or in tiny circles to clean the entire surface. Rinse with water.

- **Brush your tongue**: To remove bacteria from the tongue, brush firmly but gently from back to front. Do not go so far back in your mouth that you gag. Rinse again.

As you work to improve the health of your gums, you may notice soreness and some initial bleeding. With proper and regular brushing, these problems will disappear within one or two weeks. If the brushing is painful, please brush more gently until the soreness disappears. The bleeding will also disappear in one to two weeks; however, there is a misconception that a little bleeding of the gums is okay. Healthy gums do not bleed! This bleeding is a sign of inflammation. If it does not go away, please see your dentist.

Perhaps the best way to adapt easily to this new technique is to set up a standard routine for brushing. Brush at the same time every day, and brush your teeth in the same order every day. For example, you can brush the outer sides of your teeth from left to right across the top, and then move to the insides of your teeth and brush from right to left. Then brush the surfaces from left to right. Repeat the steps for your lower teeth. Once you get this routine down pat, you can rest assured that you have covered every area of your mouth.

You also want to be sure to:

- **Brush at least twice a day.** Make sure to brush before bed. When you sleep, your mouth gets very dry. This dryness sets up an ideal environment for acids from bacteria to attack your teeth. Also try to brush in the morning, either before or after breakfast. After breakfast is better. That way, bits of food are removed. But if you eat in your car or at work, or skip breakfast, brush first thing in the morning to get rid of the plaque that built up overnight.

- **Brush no more than three times a day.** Brushing after lunch will give you a good midday cleaning. But brushing too often can damage your gums.
- **Brush for at least two minutes.** Set a timer if you have to, but don't skimp on brushing time. Two minutes is the minimum time you need to clean all of your teeth. Many people brush for the length of a song on the radio.
- **Replace your toothbrush every three months.** Throw away your old toothbrush after three months or when the bristles start to flare, whichever comes first. If your bristles flare much sooner than every three months, you may be brushing too hard. Try easing up.

The purpose of learning to brush your teeth properly is prevention. This simple change in your daily routine can avoid irreversible damage that requires intervention with dental procedures to fix the problem. Unfortunately, in most cases of gum recession from toothbrush abrasion, the receding gums will not rebound after you stop the use of a medium or hard toothbrush. However there are treatments available to repair the damage.

The use of gum grafts (also called **Periodontal Plastic Surgery**) around these teeth may be necessary. The type of gum graft a dentist recommends may vary depending on the amount of recession a patient has, the cause of the recession, and the expected outcome of the treatment. Certain periodontal plastic surgery graft procedures can create thick tissue. This tissue will stop further recession and cover the existing unsightly root recession. However, in some cases, these procedures may not be able to cover existing recession, but can create thick tissue to stop *further* recession.

One of the most common graft procedures is the Free Gingival Graft. Historically, a thin piece of gum tissue is removed from the roof of the patient's mouth and transplanted to the graft site on the tooth. This method is effective, but requires two surgical sites. A relatively new method is the use of a freeze-dried human tissue product, commonly used in medicine for burn victims. This tissue called *"aloderm"* eliminates the need for the tissue taken from the palate of the patient's mouth. This tissue, along with new " bladeless" tunneling techniques, eliminates the surgical site on the roof of the mouth and commonly results in less post-operative discomfort. The use of *aloderm* is my method of choice when applicable, and my patients have reported little post-operative discomfort.

I hope this chapter has served as a Dental Mythbuster and convinced you that "long teeth" are not a natural result of aging. The power to prevent toothbrush abrasion literally rests in your hand. Pick up a soft toothbrush at your local pharmacy, memorize and practice the Modified Bass Brushing Technique, and see your dentist regularly.

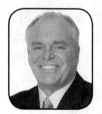

ABOUT GREG

Dr. Greg Phillips followed in his father's footsteps and became a second-generation dentist. A graduate of the Louisiana State University School of Dentistry, he has been in practice for over thirty years, and has built a large clientele based on referrals from satisfied patients. His practice now includes cosmetic, restorative, and comprehensive dentistry, with particular emphasis on tooth replacement with dental implants.

Over the years, Dr. Phillips has frequently updated his knowledge of cosmetic and restorative dentistry with continuing education courses and memberships in several highly-respected dental organizations. As a member of the International Congress of Oral Implantologists (ICOI), and a graduate of the MISCH International Implant Institute, Dr. Phillips is rapidly becoming a leader in the field of dental implants.

In addition to his fellowship at the ICOI, Dr. Phillips is also a member of the American Dental Association, the Louisiana Dental Association, and the New Orleans Dental Association.

Dr. Phillips strives to provide a comfortable atmosphere for his patients. Recognized as an expert in the area of dental office design, he has lectured extensively and authored numerous articles on the subject. Dr. Phillips has used this expertise to ensure that every patient has a pleasant dental experience at his office.

CHAPTER 5

"LIVE LONG AND PROSPER!"

BY JESSE CHAI, DDS

Yes, that is a quote from Star Trek, but its a good one. You see there has never been a better time to be alive. We know more about health and how to live longer, healthier lives than we ever have in human history. The whole purpose of this Chapter is to help you live longer and healthier by arming you with knowledge. These "secrets" will be revealed to you throughout this chapter. I am shocked how little people know about this very important body part that you use everyday and how it can affect your health. This body part is crucial for breathing, eating, drinking and communication –which are all vital for your very survival. I am of course talking about your mouth. Have you ever had a sore spot on your tongue or in your mouth, and you could not eat without pain for days? Ever have a toothache? You see, pain is a great motivator! The problem is that most things that happen in your mouth or head do not hurt or bother you until it is too late, or is so gradual that you do not perceive a true problem. So the key is to arm yourself with this top secret information, so you too can … "Live long and prosper!"

ABOUT MYSELF

Early in my career, I worked in nursing homes helping the elderly with their dental problems. I saw person after person with horrible oral hygiene, terrible teeth, and just an extreme poor state of health and well being. To make matters worse, the patients with no teeth and just dentures were in even worse shape, as the dentures never fit and they couldn't eat with them. In general, the people I saw and treated had horrible oral care, and as a result had poor nutrition. The combination of rampant bacteria in their mouth and poor nutrition was a devastating combination. I saw a number of names of people I had seen earlier in the year for assessments and simple dental work (the patients generally were not well enough to have extensive work done), deteriorate quickly and pass away. It really opened my eyes. A few years later, when I settled into my own practice, I vowed to do my best to provide my patients with the best care – so that they would avoid ending up like the poor patients I saw in the nursing homes. The reason many dentists like myself got into practice was, and is, to help people. We take many courses and are constantly learning new techniques to help our patients achieve higher levels of health.

THE SIX SECRET WAYS YOUR DENTIST CAN HELP YOU LIVE LONG AND PROSPER!

I think one of the reasons a lot of those nursing home patients I saw were in the state that they were in, was because they did not take care of their teeth when they were younger. They were too afraid to go to the dentist, or just avoided them from just indifference or procrastination, or perhaps the fear of being judged by the dentist and staff. The thing is, and I think I speak for most dentists... we are not here to judge you. Our only mission really is to help you keep your teeth for as long as you want to keep them, and to help you maintain a high quality of health for your many years to come. There are many reasons you should see your dentist regularly, and I will share with you those "Secrets", so you too can live long and prosper.

TOP SECRET #1: YOUR GUMS AND YOUR HEALTH

Did you know that gum disease has been linked to an increased risk of Heart Disease, Diabetes, certain Cancers, Stroke, and Alzheimer's? It has also been linked to premature births and low-weight babies. It has been said that 70% of the population over the age of 30 have some form of gum disease, ranging from *gingivitis* (inflammation of the gums) to advanced *periodontitis*. *Periodontitis* is the disease of the gums and bone surrounding your teeth, and is the number one cause of tooth-loss in adults. Even more shocking is that about 90% of adults over the age of 50 have some form of gum disease.

61

This is a major reason why it is crucial to take care of your gums and teeth and to see your dentist regularly. If your teeth, gums and tongue are covered with bacteria, plaque and tartar (hard plaque), you will constantly be swallowing it and the bacteria will also circulate in your blood stream. The reason we believe that gum disease is linked to an increase risk of heart disease and stroke, is that the same bacteria in your mouth is also found in the plaque around your arteries, and the only origin of these bacteria is your mouth. The bacteria in your mouth have been found in autopsies of Alzheimer patient's brains. There is a huge correlation between Diabetes and gum disease. We also know that if your body is constantly fighting infection in your mouth, which is what occurs when you have gum disease, it lowers your immune system and puts you more at risk of diseases such as certain cancers, bacterial and viral diseases.

If you only go to see the dentist every 6 months, that is 4,368 hours between professional cleanings! That is a long time. If you have gum disease, you should be seeing a dentist for a professional cleaning every 3 months, which is 2,184 hours between cleanings. Studies show that the plaque that forms on your teeth and gums starts to reform within 24 hours after your professional cleaning and has pretty much repopulated in most people within 3 months. So if you fall in the 70% of the adult population over 30, or 90% of the population of 50 that have some form of gum disease, you should consider seeing your dentist every 3 months to maintain your teeth and gums, and your long term health as well!

TOP SECRET #2:
EARLY ORAL CANCER DETECTION

As technology and screening methods have improved, so has life expectancy. Every year, women get breast exams and Pap smears, and men get prostate exams for early detection of cancer. There are now early oral cancer screening devices as well, which greatly enhance the early detection of cancer in the mouth. When oral cancer is detected early on, there is about a 90% chance of survival in 5 years. This drops to about 50% if the cancer is detected late. One of the biggest advocates of early oral cancer screenings is Colleen Zenk Pinter who played Barbara Ryan on the Soap Opera "As the World Turns." Ms. Pinter, who doesn't smoke or drink is an oral cancer survivor. There is a link between the HPV virus and Oral Cancer, so although smoking and drinking are huge risk factors, they are not the only risk factors. It is now recommended that everyone over the age of 18 should be screened once a year for oral cancer by your dentist which is just another way your dentist can help you live longer and prosper!

TOP SECRET #3:
MIGRAINES, HEADACHES, JAW PAIN, CLENCHING, GRINDING AND TMJ

This is a controversial topic so there will be dentists that disagree with this section. To describe this topic fully would require more information than this book intended. The bottom line is that if you suffer from Migraines, Headaches or Jaw Pain, it is possible that you have a disorder of your Temporomandibular Joints (TMJ) or Jaw Joints. The song, "the jaw bone is connected to the head bone, the head bone is connected to the neck bone, etc." illustrates nicely how one part of your body affects the other. When your lower jaw bone is improperly connected to your head bone, either too overclosed or too retruded, your jaw is misaligned. Your jaw muscles are also misaligned and as a result function improperly. You tend to clench and grind more to prevent the muscles from locking up – which can lead to muscle spasms. When you overwork your arm or back muscles, they go into spasm. When the head and neck muscles go into spasm, you get headaches, migraines or jaw pain. Some people even get ringing, stuffiness or even pain in their ears, and some get pain behind their eyes.

In some cases like mine, a back and neck problem can have its origins in your jaw joint. Until I had my jaw joint position corrected, my back and neck treatment was not holding. Having had six whiplash injuries over a 5-year period did a number on my neck and back, and the nature of my profession did not help. I can honestly say that without treatment of my jaw joints, my career as a dentist would have been cut short, and the quality of my life would have declined tremendously. Since everything is connected like the song above, if your jaw is out of alignment, so is the alignment of your head on your neck and spine. This was certainly the case in my situation, and I see it all too often in my practice as well.

If you are unfortunate enough to suffer from any of the following symptoms: headaches, migraines, neck or back pain, jaw pain, eye pain, ringing or stuffiness in the ears, popping or clicking in the ears, you may have a treatable TMJ issue. The more symptoms you have and especially if all other causes have been ruled out, the more likely that you have a TMJ issue, and your Dentist may be able to help. Just one more way your dentist can help you live a fuller life.

TOP SECRET #4:
BREATHING AND YOUR MOUTH

If you can imagine breathing through a very skinny straw versus a really big fat one, there is quite a difference. Your nose and mouth work in much the same way. If you have a wide mouth and nose, you can breath much easier than if you have a narrow mouth and nose. Many of you did not know that your dentist can assess and can help improve your ability to breathe! It is no secret that without oxygen you will die. There are many people that have such small mouths and noses that they can only breathe through their mouths. Now this can be due to sinus congestion or allergies, but when you add a small nose to the mix, it's hard to breathe.

Mouth breathing causes a few problems: 1). you tend to gag more easily; 2). your gums and tissues are much more red and puffy due to being dried out; 3). you have increased clenching and grinding; 4). you tend to snore more; and 5). in some people the breathing problem is so severe that you develop *sleep apnea*, where you actually stop breathing for periods at a time, which can last for minutes. Nose breathing is important for normal smooth muscle, including your heart muscle, so if you snore, it is a problem. A bigger problem is *sleep apnea*, because if you stop breathing for periods at a time, you will literally take 10 years off your life, and your quality of life will be poor.

Common symptoms of *sleep apnea* is daytime tiredness, cluster-headaches, waking up gasping for air, night time urination, and waking up tired. Football legend Reggie White and Hall of Famer Jerry Garcia of the *Grateful Dead* both died with *sleep apnea* being a contributing cause. Most highway accidents where drivers fall asleep at the wheel are *sleep apnea* related. If your child snores, they likely have *sleep apnea* and you should consult your dentist on an appropriate treatment which could include tonsil and adenoid removal by a Specialist, orthopaedic treatment (see below), allergy assessment, or all of the above.

The good news is that *sleep apnea* is treatable, and most of the time you do not need the giant compressed oxygen machine called a CPAP. You still need to be diagnosed by a physician, and usually have to go for a sleep study to confirm if you have the problem. However, the first line of defence, according to the American Association of Sleep Medicine for Mild to Moderate *sleep apnea* is an oral appliance which your dentist can make. An oral appliance is also used to treat those that refuse to wear their CPAP machine.

Another useful treatment which is especially useful in growing children, but can be done in adults in the right circumstances, is a process we call Orthopedics, which is a fancy word for bone movement. Believe it or not, the upper jaw is not one solid bone. What we have found is that when we apply light forces we can actually widen your upper jaw. This not only makes the upper jaw wider, it increases the surface area of the nose and sinus, making it easier to breath through your nose. Research has shown that for every 1mm of jaw widening, there is a 10% improvement in your ability to breathe. This works especially well on kids when they are growing, but will work on adults as well, which I can attest to. I use to have a deviated septum and had difficulty breathing though my nose. After I widened my upper jaw a little when I was going through braces later in life (early thirties), I found I no longer mouth breathe at all (unless I have a cold), and sleep more soundly than I ever have in my life. You see the reason that many dentists advocate early treatment for orthodontics on kids is that by helping to slowly develop the upper jaw, we not only create more room for the teeth, but we help your kids breathe easier as well. As a result they sleep better. As a result of sleeping better, they are able to concentrate more at school, are generally better behaved and less cranky, able to maximize growth as they are now producing more normal amounts of growth hormone, and they do not wake up in the middle of the night to go to the bathroom.

TOP SECRET #5:
YOUR TEETH AND FUNCTION

When you lose your teeth, you decrease your ability to chew. The more teeth you lose, the harder it is to enjoy your food and the poorer your nutrition becomes. As your diet worsens, you turn to more processed foods which speeds up the deterioration of your teeth and your overall health. This is why dentists work so hard to try to help you keep what you have. The reason we want you to keep your teeth is because we know how important they are for you to eat. The reason we want you to replace the teeth you lost is so you do not end up like those people I treated in the nursing homes.

Statistically, the more of your teeth you have that are functional, the longer you will live and live well, as you can eat more nutritious foods. The people that I see living into their 90s still had most or all of their natural teeth. The people I see dying in their 60s had lost most or all of their teeth, or had severe disease in their mouths. There is a huge link between the health of your teeth and your overall health. So if you have a cavity in an important tooth, and it can be saved with a filling, or a root canal and crown, do it. If you have a missing tooth and you can replace it with an implant or bridge, do it. It is to your benefit and for your long term health. Do whatever you can to save your teeth and take care of your gums. In your twilight years you will be glad you did, and you will not have any regrets as you enjoy your apple or steak.

TOP SECRET #6:
COSMETICS AND PROSPERITY

We have talked a lot about health, but what about prosperity. Cosmetic Dentistry has come along way. We can whiten your teeth, we can straighten your teeth, and we can place porcelain on your teeth to give you a gorgeous smile. The Extreme Makeover show was able to show you the power of a beautiful smile and how it can change your life.

People with bad teeth, or who are embarrassed by their smile, do not smile. People who do not smile do not get promoted and do not do well in interviews. Some people who do not like their smile can be so embarrassed that they are afraid to try anything new, and they have such low self-esteem that they feel like failures before they even start. This is an extreme example of course, but I have seen it.

I have also seen the transformation that can occur when you give someone the smile they have always wanted. It is life-changing and I have never seen anyone regret improving their smile. For some, it is truly the best investment they have even made, as their life began the day they looked at their new smile for the first time. Some people change their smile to get ahead in life, some do it for their self-esteem. Whatever the reason, if you think your smile is holding you back from being whole, your dentist can help you and would love to take that journey with you. The look on your face when you see your new smile for the first time is truly one of the best moments that occur in a dentists life. We change people's lives every day by helping them live longer by taking care of their dental needs, but rarely do we get to drastically change someone so much as to give them a new smile ...and it is a great feeling.

CONCLUSION:

Living a long, healthy and prosperous life starts with you. You need to take the initiative and go to see your dentist. As you see there are many ways that your dentist can help you, and we want to help you achieve whatever level of health you desire.

So do not delay, do not procrastinate and do not ignore your mouth. As Spock would say, "Live Long and Prosper"!

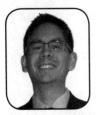

ABOUT JESSE

Dr. Jesse Chai graduated from the University of Toronto, Faculty of Dentistry in 1998. Early in his career he worked in nursing homes and around the Toronto area. It was in those nursing homes that Dr. Chai realized the true impact of improper dental care. After spending a year in Niagara Falls and Niagara-On-The Lake, he eventually settled in Bradford, Ontario, Canada. Dr. Jesse Chai is the owner and senior dentist at Bradford Family Dentistry and has been recognized for his contribution to the town of Bradford, having won the Entrepreneur of the Year award in 2006, Business Excellence award in 2010, and Customer Service Excellence Award for 2011. You can visit his website at: www.bradfordfamilydentist.ca.

Dr. Jesse Chai is committed to Excellence and has obtained more than 2000 hours of continuing education, and strongly believes in providing his patients with the best treatment he can possibly provide. His office is also committed to excellent customer service, having received live training from representatives from the Ritz Carlton and Disney Institute, as well as John DiJulius, author of "What's the Secret? To Providing a World-Class Customer Experience". Dr. Chai is committed 'to be the best he can be' and to help as many patients as he can, reach their dental health goals.

Dr. Jesse Chai enjoys running a family practice and provides many services ranging from routine Tooth Coloured fillings and cleanings to services such as Root Canals, Wisdom Tooth Removal, Implants, Dentures, Ceramic crowns and bridges, Headache and TMJ treatment, Snoring and sleep apnea treatment, Braces and Orthodontic treatment for children and adults, Cosmetic Dentistry and Veneers, and Sedation Dentistry.

Dr. Chai has incorporated a great deal of technology into his practice to also help him provide what he feels is better services to his patients. The technology Dr. Chai chooses to incorporate serves three main functions:

1. better diagnostic ability for prevention,

2. better ability to show patients what is occurring in their mouths so

they can make informed decisions regarding their dental care and

3. saving the patients time by using technology to provide more efficient care.

He uses intra-oral cameras and digital cameras to help patients see what is happening in their mouths. He uses digital x-rays to reduce the patient's radiation exposure and also allows patients to see more easily what is occurring in their mouths as images can be blown up to the size of the computer screen. He uses an in-office crown-making machine called Cerec AC which allows patients to receive Porcelain crowns and fillings in one office visit which greatly cuts down on office visits and the patient's time away from work. Dr. Chai also uses laser technology for more rapid tissue healing and gum tissue treatment. He also uses a special cavity-detecting laser called a Diagnodent to help find cavities at their earliest stages. He uses an Oral Cancer Screening device called a Velscope to help detect oral cancer at the earliest stages. Dr. Chai also uses electric motors to reduce drilling times in the mouth, and rapid-curing lights that can harder your fillings in as little as one second. This greatly reduces the time to place your fillings, and helps reduce the time you are in the dentist's chair!

Your comfort is another area of technology Dr. Chai has invested in, with Memory foam padded dental chairs, and some chairs with massage and heat functions. There are also TV's in each treatment room for your entertainment while you receive your dental care.

Dr. Chai is married and has one young son who he enjoys hanging out with at home. Dr. Chai also enjoys reading and learning. He is passionate about self-improvement, and is often found listening to audio programs on his iPod, watching educational videos on his computer, or traveling and attending live events. Dr. Chai enjoys watching TV and movies with his wife.

For more information on Dr. Chai and his practice, go to:
www.bradfordfamilydentist.ca

CHAPTER 6

THE MOMENT OF TRUTH:
HOW THE PATIENT EXPERIENCE CAN BE A LIFE-SAVER

BY MARK FIXARI, DDS

"Cure sometimes, treat often, comfort always. "

~ Hippocrates

What's the critical moment of truth in any relationship? *In my opinion, it's that all-important first meeting* – when you initially judge just how much you can trust the other person and how comfortable you feel around them. Generally, unless you've heard something extremely negative or positive about that person in advance, you make those judgments based on your intuition and gut feeling – and it can be difficult, moving forward, to overcome those initial feelings.

And it's no different with doctors and patients. In the typical healthcare experience, your initial moment with the doctor is the moment of truth. And it's no different with any member of your practice staff – *every* interaction is critical to establishing a crucial bond of trust with a patient.

In my own dental practice, as well as in my coaching of other dentists and dental teams, this is a concept I make sure to emphasize. Of course, the actual care of a patient is a critical and important matter - but getting that patient to trust you and put him or herself into your care is the vital first step towards that care-giving as well as its ultimate success. Research and studies back up this notion – and I'd like to illustrate just how important it is through a compelling real-life story in which I'm incredibly proud to be a participant.

There are people out there we call "avoiders" – dental phobics who just can't bring themselves to have their teeth examined. This can obviously lead to some dangerous situations – and the story I'm about to tell you is the most extreme one with which I've ever been involved.

RON'S STORY

Some years ago, Ron, the patient that this story is about, was at a baseball game with his brother-in-law, who was a patient of mine. After a couple of beers, Ron loosened up – and started telling his brother-in-law that he had a great deal of pain in his mouth, but that he was afraid to see a dentist about the problem. A little later, he began to tell him that his whole life had been affected by his extreme fear of dentists. He was a National Sales Manager, but couldn't do his job as well as he should, because he was uncomfortable with the appearance of his teeth – and it was the same with his marriage, which was now over. His mouth issues had been a big factor in his divorce.

His brother-in-law told him flat out that he couldn't go on like this. He needed to go see the dentist – and he recommended me. He told him about how our practice treated patients very well and that we would treat him in the best and most reassuring way possible. Ron, however, couldn't make an appointment – he still couldn't overcome his fear.

The problem was that he also couldn't overcome the growing pain in his mouth, which was becoming unbearable. After some more coaxing from his brother-in-law, Ron finally got our number and gave us a call. He still didn't want to come in, but our receptionist was so warm and friendly (part of our overall people-first approach), that he was convinced to finally make an appointment.

He lived a good distance from our practice, but made the big drive for his scheduled visit. When he arrived, he was still nervous and reluctant. We had cookies and coffee to put him more at ease, but he still said he would not submit to any treatment. He wouldn't even sit in the patient chair – so this was not going to be easy!

Finally, he allowed us to take a Panorex X-Ray, because, for that device, nothing had to be put in his mouth. For those of you who aren't familiar with a Panorex X-ray, it's done with a machine that literally travels around your head and takes an X-ray of your complete upper and lower jaw.

Well, since he had not been to the dentist in years and years – basically his entire adult life – his teeth were hopeless. Beyond that, we were very concerned about one particular area in the X-ray.

Luckily, because we were gentle with him and treated him with respect, he allowed us to do some work. We sent out for a biopsy on the problem area we had targeted. We also had the oral surgeon we work with put him under with anesthetic, take molds and put in some immediate dentures.

Well, he came back in a few days after the surgery, grinning ear-to-ear. He was a completely different guy – his new teeth gave him confidence as well as an enormous sense of relief from having addressed a major problem that was affecting his entire life in a very negative way.

Unfortunately, what Ron didn't know yet, was that the biopsy revealed that he had squamous-cell carcinoma, a very deadly form of oral cancer with a poor five-year survival rate. So we had to sit him down and tell him about the horrible prognosis 'and puncture his happy balloon.'

This was one of the most significant moments I've ever had as a professional. His newfound joy was completely destroyed and he was sobbing like a baby. Ron had remarried since his divorce, and we called his new wife over to help him get home.

While we were waiting for her, he calmed down and asked what the next step was. We told him we had arranged for him to see a cancer specialist at Ohio State in a few weeks. You may have heard of Dr. Kübler-Ross's five stages of grief – well, I had already witnessed Ron go through a few of them and now he transitioned to Anger. He was upset that he had to wait that long and started yelling about how it was unacceptable. He was very intimidating, but eventually once again regained his composure and even managed to get an appointment with the specialist a little sooner on his own.

I continued to worry about Ron, and, a few weeks later, I took my eight year-old son to the Ohio State football game. At halftime, we walked over to the cancer center, where I knew he was being treated. And that treatment was quite severe, especially for a man who feared anything being done to his mouth. Half of his jaw had to be removed and it was replaced with part of his shinbone. I was a little concerned about what his mental state might be after going through all of that and knowing his chances of beating the cancer weren't great.

We went up to the floor on which he was being treated and, as we came down the hall, I could spot his room easily – his room was filled with people that he had been watching the game with. We entered and I saw him laying in bed with numerous tubes attached to him for various medical needs.

He could barely talk – his voice was quite hoarse from all the procedures – and, as I said, he was connected to a lot of machinery. Nevertheless, when he saw me, he stood up with a great deal of difficult – then he looked at me, then turned to at all the people in the room and croaked out, "This is the man who saved my life."

And then he began crying as he hugged me. …And kept hugging me. …And kept sobbing.

It was incredibly moving – but I could only think that I didn't really *do* anything for him. I didn't do the surgery that gave him the new teeth. I didn't diagnose the cancer or treat it. The only thing I had done for him was deal with him as a *person* who desperately needed help – and to create the kind of practice where even someone as frightened of dentists as he was, could conquer that fear and build a bond of trust with my staff. And, looking back on it, it was the focus of everyone in my practice on the overall patient experience that saved his life – that was all I could really take credit for.

You may be wondering what happened to Ron. Well, thankfully, he has survived the cancer – and, since it has been over five years with no recurrence, he has an excellent chance of living a long and healthy life. We put dental implants in his mouth and gave him a completely cosmetic makeover – and there's no procedure he'll say "no" to now!

And there was one more small side benefit to my personal life, since my son witnessed Ron's heartfelt thank you to me. Later on, when one of his friends found out what his dad did for a living, said to him, "Your dad's a dentist? That's the easiest job in the world!" Boy, did my son have a story to tell him!

Putting people first pays off both on a professional and personal level. I'm thankful that it not only works so well for my practice, but that I'm also able to help other dental professionals deliver the same kind of awesome patient experience in their practices.

PUTTING PEOPLE FIRST

Now I'd like to explain more about our approach at Fixari Family Dental (and when we say *"Family* Dental," we mean it – my wife Shayne is also a dentist and the real brains of the operation, plus we have seven kids!).

To understand that approach, you first have to understand the reason we bake chocolate cookies at our practice every day.

Most people are nervous about going to the dentist, that's nothing new. And one of the big things that sets them on edge is just the *smell* of the typical dental practice. That's where the cookies come in. When you come into a dental office and smell chocolate chips baking…well, that's a whole different experience. You think of home, instead of drills and spit sinks.

We've all faced fear and pain in a health care environment – I've had my own experiences when I was diagnosed with and treated for melanoma some years back. What I feel medical professionals and their staffs really need to do is to key in on how they *themselves* have felt in the past, when having those kinds of fear-filled experiences. That helps them to empathize with patients – and to know what to do in order to help those patients feel more comfortable when they come in for an appointment.

The most important part of a practice's experience with a patient is relationship building. Everyone who goes to see the doctor or the dentist has similar questions in their mind – "Am I important to them?" …"Do they want to understand me and help me?" And everyone is unconsciously answering those questions at every turn as they go through a practice's process.

I always say that when a patient is sitting in the reception area, they're not really reading the magazines – they're taking in what's going on. They're listening to how the phone is answered, they're listening to how other patients are both being greeted and said goodbye to, and they're listening to the sounds coming from examination rooms. If they pick up a negative atmosphere from all that, it's going to make them feel jumpy, nervous and anxious.

That's why we work as hard as we can, in every aspect of our practice, to make our patients feel as 'at home' as possible. For a dentist, fixing teeth can get to be a bore, but people never do. When your focus is on the patients and creating the best experience you can, that never gets old – because every person is different and has different needs.

Believe me, when you do apply this focus, it doesn't just benefit the patient, it also benefits your practice and your business. When people are really taken care of, they respond by staying with you and recommending you to their friends and family members. And, in my case, it even opened up a whole new business.

My best friend is an accountant who has over a hundred other dentists who were clients. He always admired how we ran our practice, so, when he would get a client who was fairly new to dentistry, he would ask me if that person could follow me around and see how I did things. I was glad to help out at first, but it got to the point where I just didn't have the time to run the practice and show these dentists the ropes. That's when my accountant had a brilliant idea – that I should set up a coaching business for dentists and dental teams on the side.

So that's just what I did, and it's something I really enjoy. But, more than that, I feel great about the patients I've helped through my "people-first" approach. And one patient, more than any other, really validated that approach to a degree I never thought possible.

No matter what your business might be, having a focus on people can't help but be beneficial. After all…people are what it's all about!

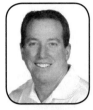

ABOUT MARK

Mark and Shayne Fixari founded Fixari Family Dental in the fall of 1987 with a vision to change the perception of a typical dental office. This compassionate approach brings many of their patients from far away. The dentists at Fixari Family Dental are all members of the American Dental Association, Ohio Dental Association, Columbus Dental Society and Central Ohio Study Club.

Dr. Mark's passion for the artistic aspect of life-changing cosmetic dentistry is fueled by unending energy for continuing education. Dr. Shayne loves to give her young and old patients special attention in a very caring, empathetic environment. Having seven children of their own, they have created an atmosphere children and adults have come to really appreciate.

Drs. Fixari now spend a significant amount of time writing, speaking and educating other dentists and dental offices on creating an exceptional, patient-centered experience.

Dr. Mark Fixari is a member of the Board of Directors of the Columbus Dental Society.

CHAPTER 7

HOW TO KEEP YOUR TEETH FOREVER!
— OR SEVEN KEYS TO A HAPPY MOUTH!

BY ROY WRATHER, DDS

Have you ever had a tooth ache? Have you ever been embarrassed with your smile, holding your hand over your mouth as you talk? Have you wondered if your breath was fresh or reminded people of a dead animal? Have you had to spend money you didn't want to spend, or to spend time in a less than fun manner?

Let me tell you how to keep your teeth in a practical way. There are many different ideas regarding these problems and solutions. People are always asking me how to avoid me (the dentist). How about that? I will show you how to not have to see me and keep your teeth.

I get my greatest joy by helping people to stop needing me very much. I don't want my patients to redo the same fillings over and over, then give up and get dentures, and all the trouble that accompanies that scenario. I get a kick out of these patients getting to do the fun things in dentistry like cosmetic dentistry in all its forms, like veneers, crowns, orthodontics, and replacement therapy, including implants. I really enjoy helping people look good, feel good, eat good, smell good, taste good and have the security of knowing they have a healthy mouth.

If I want to go on vacation to Florida, lie in the sand and eat lots of seafood, I first look at a map so I could get there by the most efficient route possible. I could then spend my time enjoying the beach instead of driving around aimlessly looking for a 'fun bunch of sand.' Likewise, my patients should first have a thorough examination to find out their condition. Then, if there is any disease – i.e., periodontitis (gum infection), tooth decay (tooth infection) or jawbone infection, we could then deal with it appropriately. If there was a condition like missing, crooked or discolored teeth, we would also be able to do the same. Desires of the patients need to be dealt with. Sometimes a patient comes in who has had a burning desire for a long time. They may not have dealt with it because of hopelessness, perhaps because their parents lost their teeth, or they have had to refill a cavity many times, because there was no plan to heal the infection.

Now we know the present condition. We can now make a plan for success. Usually the first thing to do is to stop the worsening problems of gum infection and tooth decay. Gum infection is highly implicated with diabetes, strokes and some types of heart attacks. Most premature tooth loss is due to gum infection. Wow! That makes it sound important, does it not? Well it is. Of course, everyone knows that tooth decay leads to horrific pain, abscesses, bad-smelling breath, and ugly teeth!

What causes all this destruction? What can we do about it ourselves to stop the ravages of oral infection? We are lucky. Dr. C. C. Bass at Loyola University in 1919 discovered the secret. Surprisingly, it still seems to be a secret today. This is the entire foundation of effective, efficient, affordable dentistry. This plan works better than any other methodology. This really is a biofilm problem. Drilling and filling the cavities is not sufficient treatment because this disease itself needs to be identified and treated. If not, the area will just re-decay around the filling until it gets so bad it is lost, or if we again intervene early enough to save the tooth.

So, what do you do?

Let us look at a normal mouth like the ones I may see every day. Lets assume that our patient, lets call him Roger, has just had a very thorough cleaning and polishing to get his teeth just right. Well, in just twenty-four hours, something very amazing has happened in Roger's mouth. The very, very few bacteria left behind after the professional cleaning begin to multiply! These types of bacteria multiply by mitosis. Mitosis is cell division. It is the process by which a cell divides into two daughter cells, each of which has the same number of chromosomes as the original cell. It is just one bacterium splitting down the middle. Now there are two. It happens again. Now there are four. ... Now eight. ...Now sixteen. ...Now thirty two. You can see that if this happens in seconds, then in twenty-four hours there will be millions/billions of bacteria in the mouth. They are hiding under the gums, between the teeth, and by now even on the open surfaces of the teeth.

The story is like this. The little nasty germs that live between your teeth, under your gums and down in the little groove on your teeth, love sugar just as you do. Here is the problem. When the germs in your mouth eat the sugars that you have just eaten – it gives them diarrhea!!!! Now the germs begin to die and rot. So now, you have piles of dead rotting bacteria covered in "bug doo" and you wonder why breath smells bad sometimes?

That sticky pile of dead bacteria covered in bug doo is called plaque. Quite a benign name for such an awful thing, don't you think? If you were to look very closely at that plaque with a special type of microscope called a phase microscope, you would see a very interesting story. Suppose you got your teeth cleaned very well on day one, you would not see very much through that microscope. By the end of the first day, you would see scattered clumps of little round **cocci** *bacteria. These clumps are colonies of bacteria. These are strep-type organisms. This type of colony produces very weak acids and toxins. It takes twenty four hours for the colony to coalesce into the clump of bacteria. If you don't disturb this colony even in one place on your tooth for three days, you begin to see a growth of* **diplococcus** *organisms. They make stronger acids and toxins. After five days, rod-shaped organisms appear, producing even stronger and stronger acids and toxins. Seven days brings filamentous organisms with the same acid and toxin increase. Finally, after fourteen days of undisturbed plaque, you see spirochetes! Oh, no!*

When the colony consolidates with the protective covering of aerobic (with oxygen) bacteria and the bad anaerobic (without oxygen) bacteria underneath where oxygen cannot get to them, they in turn leave behind very toxic and acidic remains. These soft, sticky, squirmy, nasty, smelly destructive agents begin to <u>break down the gum tissue</u> *and* <u>dissolve the tooth enamel</u>*. This destroys the skin covering the gums in the little groove (sulcus) around the tooth, and there is nothing to hold the blood in. There is also nothing to keep the germs out of the gum tissue. That is what skin does. It keeps the blood in and the germs out.*

It is just like if you cut your arm. It would bleed and germs would get into the cut. It might get infected and hurt, swell up, fill with pus, infect your blood stream and then you die! Well most of the time it isn't so bad. However, at the very least you have heard stories of this happening after all sorts of accidents. So, you clean the site and possibly put medications on it. You might even put a band-aid or some kind of sterile dressing on it. It is a little difficult to put a band-aid on the inside of your gums. It bleeds if you touch it by brushing or probing with a measuring instrument. That is how you know that the gum is infected. It also looks deeper red and sometimes turns almost blue. Sometimes, infections in the mouth, just like anywhere else, get very serious. There has been a lot of press lately about soft, sticky, squirmy, nasty, smelly gum disease (periodontitis) being implicated in all sorts of problems like strokes, diabetes and some types of heart attacks.

Your soft, sticky, squirmy, nasty, smelly plaque germ colony gets to the point where all of the different bacteria live in a symbiotic relationship. (Symbiotic = mutually beneficial relationship; i.e., a close association of animals or plants of different species that is often of mutual benefit.) The first rather innocuous germs form a coating that protects the deeper more dangerous germs.

These spirally-mobile bad guys are anaerobic. This means that they live only in the absence of oxygen. Each of the succeeding previously mentioned bacterial colonies lives on less and less oxygen as the poisons gets stronger and stronger. If you ever see a sewage treatment vat, you may notice a big stirring rod going round and round. This rod's purpose is to stir oxygen into the liquid. When oxygen gets to the worst bacteria, they die.

There is left behind a hard tightly-attached material called calculus or tartar. I do not know why there are two names for the same thing. I guess that is just how the world is. Anyway, we will call it calculus. That sounds like some complicated math problem, doesn't it? If you were to pull out the old microscope again and look at this material, it looks like coral. You know, like the coral from the ocean. Think about it. How would you clean coral if it had soft, sticky, squirmy, nasty, smelly bacteria colonies on it. It would look like "Goo" on the coral. You know, that soft, sticky, squirmy, nasty, smelly green stuff kids play with. You are totally grossed out again, so I will continue. Obviously, you will not be able to remove all that hard and soft stuff from your teeth and gums yourself.

You may be tempted to clean your own teeth, but I assure you that you will not do a good job and you will damage your own teeth. The hygienist must do it. The hygienist will have many special instruments both electronic and steel that fit the complicated curvy surfaces of your teeth just right. These health professionals have been highly trained to do this very specialized treatment. When they talk about "gum treatment", they are referring to cleaning out the diseased tissue of the gum and removing all the calculus and smoothing all surfaces of the tooth so it is smooth and slick. Now it is slick and smooth and you can clean it daily with home instruments. The first thing you do is brush as much plaque off as you can with the toothbrush. The second thing is to floss the areas between your teeth to remove the plaque (soft, sticky, squirmy, nasty, smelly bacteria colonies).

So, again, what do you do?

SEVEN KEYS TO A HAPPY MOUTH (WITH TEETH!)

1. Commit to keeping your teeth. Commit your time, your energy, your focus and your money. Without serious commitment, all goals fail. You must know why you want to accomplish this goal and have a written and dated step-plan that will.
2. Commit to learning the existing condition, causes, cures and solutions for your mouth.
3. Commit to a caring, focused, preventive-oriented Dentist with a good local reputation for excellence. Make sure and find one who will communicate his findings clearly to you in a manner you understand. Ask your friends. Check the phonebook, other media, billboards, and the dental staff. The staff may give you good insight into the type of dentist and the type of person the dentist is.
4. Commit to an appointment for an initial examination. Ask what will be done. Ask, in

detail, how long it is and why it is so important to start with the examination. Then, just make the appointment. Just do it! Go with trust and anticipation of being well cared for.

5. Commit to listening carefully to the words of the dentist and the hygienist or assistant who works with the dentist. When the examination is finished, you should have a good idea of all the problems in your mouth and neck. The solutions may take a little longer to discover. Sometimes to find out what your next treatment needs to be, some initial treatment must first be performed. It often depends on just how sick your teeth or gums are. Do not forget you are committed to keeping your teeth for a lifetime! The big five questions concern your comfort, beauty, pleasing breath and taste, and efficient enjoyable chewing, as well as giving you the security of knowing you have a healthy mouth functioning well. With your input, the dentist will make such a plan.

6. Commit to homecare. The most important thing of all is homecare. Nothing even comes close to doing as much for the health of your mouth. Homecare consists of brushing, flossing, irrigating, and possibly using another instrument also designed to remove plaque. A diet filled with sugars and acids makes the likelihood of ongoing success disappear. You can do more or the professional team can do more, whatever it takes for success.

7. Commit to periodic checkups. The second most important thing is having the dentist or hygienist periodically examine your mouth carefully and clean your teeth and gums. The period of time between, and the intensity of your visits, will

depend on many things. It will depend on the severity of the initial condition of your teeth and gums, how much has been repaired and/ or replaced, your motivation and skill with your homecare, your genetics and your diet.

So, there it is. Go and do it!

ABOUT ROY

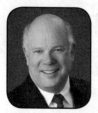

Dr. Roy Wrather has emerged as a stalwart in today's world of Total Modern Dentistry combined with 'old world' artisanship and charm. As an entertaining, lively and provocative guest, he has appeared on TV talks shows sharing his ideas about the realities of dentistry.

Determined to practice a preventive model of dentistry where patients could have real hope of healing or controlling the diseases that ravage mouths (and by extension the entire body), and causing pain, embarrassment, time loss and energy loss.

Dr. Wrather studied undergrad at Rhodes College in Memphis, and then graduated with a Math and Physical Sciences major at Memphis University. After that, he attended the University of Tennessee Medical units in Memphis, and received his Doctor of Dental Surgery Degree.

Awards: Dr. Wrather was awarded the Richard Doggett Dean and Margaret Taylor Dean award and the Dental Auxiliary Utilization award from The University of Tennessee Medical Units at Memphis Dental School. He received The Patron of the Year, and the Man of the Year, from civic organizations in Covington.

After a short stint with the public health department in central Missouri, he set up private practice in Covington, TN. This is a small town in West Tennessee just south of Memphis. Covington is a cross between a John Grisham and Rosemunde Pilcher-book town, with all the charm and intrigue that is inherent in such a town. This town has turned out to be a good place to have the type of practice Dr. Wrather desired, and to raise his daughters.

Dr. Wrather has his dream practice that emphasizes preventive dentistry and co-diagnosis, along with treatment planning with the patient who is usually already a friend.

He still has his practice and resides there with his wife Brenda. Dr. Wrather and Brenda are active in the town and their church. Their four daughters and nine grandchildren live close in Covington and Memphis.

To learn more about Dr. Wrather and his practice, go to:
www.wratherdentalcenter.com

CHAPTER 8

DENTISTRY MAKES A DIFFERENCE

BY CLIFFORD BROWN, DDS

Most people don't view going to the dentist as a life-changing experience. They show up for their regular cleanings, get fillings as needed and generally enjoy good oral health. That's because they do come in on a regular basis – so we're able to spot problems before they get too serious. Those problems can usually be taken care of easily, efficiently and inexpensively – because they are still in the beginning stages.

The irony is that, when you never experience major dental problems, it can be easy to take what your dentist does for granted. If you see the dentist for your regularly scheduled appointments, you can generally avoid more advanced and painful issues with your teeth and gums. You're able to chew your food well and maintain your health with all the valuable nutrients those foods have to offer.

When you don't see the dentist for some time, however, you open yourself up to a lot of health risks. You have no idea what's going on in your mouth until it's too late – because there's usually no pain involved when disease is in process. You can end up missing work due to a tooth-ache. Advanced gum disease also creates a bigger chance for strokes and heart disease, as well as limits your abil-ity to fight-off infections. And did you know that pregnant women with poor oral hygiene have a greater chance of delivering babies with low birth weights?

Quality of life also suffers. Bad breath, and of course dis-colored and missing teeth, cause people to avoid social situations that might be embarrassing; that has incredibly negative effects on both their careers and personal relation-ships. They also end up not smiling and even covering their mouth with their hands, because they're ashamed of the way their teeth look.

That's why dentistry does make a big difference. It's vi-tally important to our overall well-being both physically and psychologically. The only way to really understand the power of that difference, however, is through the eyes of someone who, for one reason or another, has avoided get-ting the dental treatment they desperately needed for a long period of time.

That's why, in this chapter, I'd like to share the stories of three of my patients, who literally had their lives trans-formed by allowing their dental issues to finally be ad-dressed. Those serious problems were preventing them from living life to the fullest – and they all found a happy ending when they were resolved. I have changed each of their names to protect their privacy.

NO LAUGHING MATTER

Can you imagine a stand-up comic that doesn't feel comfortable smiling?

Don showed up in my treatment chair about a week before Christmas. Unlike many patients who avoided dentists for an extended period of time, he wasn't nervous about coming in for an appointment; he just no longer trusted dentists.

When I looked into his mouth, I soon knew why that was the case. Don had broken a few of his front teeth over the years. Now there were spaces between his front teeth and, horrifyingly, a big oversized white crown over his right front tooth, sitting almost directly under the middle of his nose. You couldn't help but stare at it – which is why Don didn't smile and hid his teeth while he spoke.

And yes, Don used to do stand-up comedy at night. He stopped performing when he began to be afraid of being heckled about his front teeth. He was still a salesman by day, but, of course, his dental problems affected that job as well. He had to deal directly with customers and was embarrassed every moment he had to spend time with them – not the best mindset for a salesman. The final straw was that, because he hadn't been to a dentist in some time, he was in pain from tooth decay and was having difficulty sleeping. After hearing his story, I could feel his pain myself.

Fortunately, since he had been a comic, he had old head-shots of himself back when his smile was still handsome

– so I had a good idea of what his front teeth should look like. I began by performing a series of examinations on him to determine the state of his oral health, and took a set of full mouth X-rays.

I determined Don needed endodontic therapy (i.e. a root canal) on the tooth that was causing him pain. Study models were taken and we decided we would need to do a four-tooth fixed-bridge to fix his smile. I took more impressions and an occlusal record to replicate how Don brought his teeth together. I sent all of these, including his old head shot, to my lab to make a provisional (temporary) bridge.

When Don returned the next week, I treated the badly decayed tooth by completing endodontic therapy and a crown buildup. I also prepped the other three front teeth and took an impression of them as well. When I finished the process, I cemented the four tooth provisional bridge into place. Don found that it all felt strange to him – he was used to having those big spaces between his teeth - but he was happy with the look.

That happiness peaked when I inserted the final restorations. He took a look in the mirror and beamed at his new smile, saying the words every dentist wants to hear – "That's better than what I was hoping for." His entire outlook on life changed for the better, and his self-esteem was back where it needed to be. Thanks to the treatment, this comic got his smile back – and was soon back on stage.

GETTING HIS BITE BACK

Steve, as opposed to Don, was already my patient and had been for a few years. However, he was like Don in that he wasn't nervous about seeing the dentist – although he did ask for nitrous oxide ("laughing gas") to relax him when he was having dental work done. And, also like Don, he had a front tooth that was in a lot of pain and would require a root canal.

That front tooth wasn't in pain from neglect, though – it was from overwork. You see, Steve was missing a lot of his back teeth – as a matter of fact, he didn't have one back tooth that had another tooth opposite to it. That meant Steve could not chew at all with his back teeth – he could only chew with his front teeth, which had caused most of them to be worn down to the gum line.

Not only that, but some of his side teeth had grown longer because there were no teeth opposite them to keep them the length they should be. As you can imagine, Steve's smile was not exactly one to admire. So he had learned to smile without actually opening his lips.

Also, unfortunately, the loss of all those back teeth had caused a lot of bone loss, causing his face to sag and making him appear much older than he actually was.

Why hadn't I treated all this before? Because Steve had had removable appliances made for him in the past to try and fix the problem – but he hated using them and refused to allow me to attempt any other solutions. He only allowed me to treat whatever was a problem at the moment – so I had to satisfy myself with just putting out fires.

Even now, when it was clear his ability to chew with his remaining teeth was in danger, he only wanted to have the root canal done on the tooth that was in pain.

I did treat the tooth, but I also asked him to return in two weeks. I was determined to find a solution to both his smile's appearance and his chewing issues. Knowing the seriousness of the situation, he was ready to let me try.

Looking over his x-rays and study models, I thought about his case. Implants, the logical solution, were out of the question due to the cost, as well as the fact that he didn't have enough bone left in his mouth for proper attachment. That took me back to using removable appliances, which Steve had already rejected.

In order to find different options, I took all of Steve's information to a prosthodontist, which is a dentist who specializes in replacing missing teeth and other structures, in order to restore the patient's appearance, comfort and health. I also took his study models to a seminar being held by one of the leading dental experts. Both agreed that removable appliances would have to be used, in conjunction with fixed crowns.

Now I had to convince Steve. I explained how this system would be better than the removable appliances he had used before. We would need to treat both his upper and lower arches at the same time, and use provisional appliances for a while to get his jaw muscles used to the new bite. Steve asked a lot of questions – How long would the treatment take? How much would it cost? ...etc. Finally he agreed to start the treatment.

After two more appointments, Steve had a complete set of provisionals – and a whole new personality. He wasn't close-lipped anymore – now he always flashed a big, broad smile and his natural warmth and confidence was allowed to come to the surface. The treatment was successful and Steve was a new man.

HIDING FROM THE WORLD

My final story, and one of the most extreme ones, began on a Tuesday, where we faced a strange situation. Our dental office was suffering a partial power outage – our compressors, suction machine and computers were all out of commission as a result. Our hall lights were out as well, but our treatment room lights still worked, so I was able to do consultations.

This was probably not a great time for John to come into our offices for the first time. Actually, it was a minor miracle that he had come in at all.

John was a very nervous middle-aged man who was obviously trying to control his anxiety. I sat down next to him and began to speak to him as gently as possible, because it was clear he would spook easily. I soon found out that he struggled with Agoraphobia, which, if you don't know, is the fear of leaving one's home and encountering other people and/or being in strange places. That struggle had cost him his many former friends as well as a thriving business. Now, his world had shrunk to the point where he would only venture out to a few familiar locations, one of them being his therapist's office.

Then we got to the really scary part – for me anyway. He had not been to a dentist in over thirty years.

As a result, he had many broken and infected teeth. And, since he also had diabetes, he was afraid he was a walking time bomb. He wanted his infected teeth gone – and to have a new, natural-looking smile instead.

After reviewing his medical history and doing a thorough examination, I called John to discuss my treatment plan for him – which presented one big, immediate problem. His gums were obviously a disaster area and we would need to get him back to our dental office to see the periodontist who works with us. Returning to our office and meeting with yet another stranger was a challenge – comparable to climbing Mount Everest to John.

He paused a moment, and then finally agreed to come back for the follow-up appointment with the periodontist. Frankly, I was far from certain he would actually return – but return he did. His eyes still betrayed his fear as he walked down our hall slowly and hesitantly to the treatment room – but he seemed just a bit more confident than last time and had more of a sense of accomplishment. He was clearly proud that he had managed the inner strength to come back – and excited that he was finally doing something about the severe condition of his teeth.

Although we did use I.V. sedation when we extracted his diseased teeth, his subsequent dental appointments went without a hitch – and he didn't seem to mind the treatment at all. As a matter of fact, he seemed somewhat happy about going through all the procedures. After all his work was completed, the healing process went smoothly, and only a few minor adjustments to his bite were needed. He adapted to his new appliances quickly.

Despite the fact that everything had gone well, I still never expected what I saw three months after he had been in the office for his last appointment. It was a few days before Christmas and I suddenly heard John's voice at the front desk. I came out and saw him standing there with gifts and thank you cards for myself, our periodontist and our entire staff.

I couldn't believe my eyes – he was like an entirely different person. He had always been hunched over like the shy scared person he was – but now, he was standing erect with a big, wide smile, a smile I was happy to have given him. His handshake was confident and firm. He had clearly made a giant leap forward in how he had perceived himself and he looked about ten years younger.

All I could think to myself was, "Mission accomplished."

Yes, dentistry can make a big difference in people's lives, as these stories demonstrate. All three of these people went through a lot of pain – and I'm not just talking about physical pain. They also suffered psychological trauma that affected them adversely, both personally and professionally.

Dentists are here to help – and we've developed many new tools not only to put patients at ease, but also to treat the most severe dental issues. If you're nervous about going to see a dentist, do yourself a favor. Get a recommendation on a good dentist from a friend or family member, make an appointment and discuss your concerns with him or her.

Make a difference in your life!

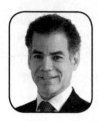

ABOUT CLIFF

Gentle Hands, warm heart. Treating you like family. A philosophy on which Dr. Clifford Brown has based his practice and his methodology of practicing Dentistry for almost 30 years.

Dr. Cliff Brown first opened the doors of Babylon Dental Care in January of 1983 with the intention of treating each and every patient as they would the members of their own family. Throughout the years, he has excelled and earned recognition and great respect for upholding this vision.

With a Bachelor of Science degree in Biology from American University in 1973, Dr. Brown went on to obtain his D.D.S. degree from SUNY at Buffalo. From the moment he opened his first practice, Dr. Brown earned a reputation for being professional, caring and sincere, with a kind, gentle nature. He has a gift for putting a patient at ease, allowing one to walk away with a positive dental experience.

Dr. Brown is always expanding his knowledge of dentistry and keeping up with the latest techniques. His continuing education includes courses in cosmetic dentistry, endodontic therapy, implant dentistry and practice management. Dr. Brown is a member of the Dental Organization for Conscious Sedation (DOCS), the New York Dental Association, Suffolk County Dental Society, and the American Dental Association.

Outside of the office, Dr. Brown loves spending time with his wife, children and circle of friends. He is well known in the community and can be found enjoying golf, baseball, traveling, and his Tuesday night card game with friends he has known since kindergarten.

To learn more about Dr. Brown or his thriving practice, visit: www.babylondentalcare.com

CHAPTER 9

"THEY ARE NOT JUST BABY TEETH"

-10 THINGS YOU CAN DO TO ADD TEN YEARS TO YOUR CHILD'S LIFE

BY WILLIAM DONHISER, DDS

D r. Charles Mayo of the Mayo Clinic once said, "If a person can take care of their teeth and gums they can extend their life by at least 10 years." Most parents or prospective parents can probably agree that they would do anything humanly possible to add an additional ten years to their child's life. What if you could work towards the goal of adding ten years to your child's life before they were even born?

To that end, by age two years you will most likely have gotten your child a series of as many as 24 vaccines to keep him or her healthy. You know that the best gift you can give your child is a long, healthy life. But do you realize that taking care of their mouth can help do that? Do you realize that dental disease is the single most prevalent disease in our country? It is five times more common than asthma and four times more common than childhood obesity!

To begin with, there are a couple things you can do *before* your child is born, or conceived for that matter, to safeguard your child's dental health – establish good eating and nutritional habits for yourself and your spouse and get your own dental house in order. Getting proper vitamins and minerals during pregnancy is essential for both the mother's and the baby's overall health. How? Poor nutrition in pregnancy can affect bone and tooth formation. The greatest gift you can give your child dentally is to take care of yourself first with proper nutrition and oral hygiene. Folic acid, calcium, and other vitamins and minerals have been proven to aid the developing fetus. A mother should have her own dental health in order before and during pregnancy. When a child is born they do not have the bacteria present that cause cavities, but contact with the 'evil' bacteria can come all too quickly. "Bad" bacteria in a child's mouth comes in innocent ways, such as mom sharing a spoon or a straw with the child or by blowing on the child's food to cool it -- which is actually transferring the bacteria to the child's mouth. This may be part of the myth of why if mom has dental decay, the child is assumed to be going to have bad teeth!

When the baby arrives you should keep these things in mind:

1. *Decay is not hereditary.* Many people believe that decay is hereditary, this is false. The bacteria that cause tooth decay are not present in a newborn's

mouth but are introduced as a child interacts with his environment. Bacteria that cause decay often are passed from caregiver to child which leads to the "I had bad teeth, my child has bad teeth, it runs in my family" falsehood.

2. *It's not okay to fall asleep while eating.* Do not let your child fall asleep breast-feeding or bottle-feeding. Also, a baby should be off breast or bottle by 10-12 months of age.

3. *Sugar is not bad.* Infants need the calories sugar provides to grow. It is not the amount of sugar that your child consumes that is the problem. It is the amount of time the teeth are exposed to decay-causing sugars that is critical.

4. *Babies do need dentists.* Your child should see a dentist for his or her first visit by six months or when their first tooth appears. The American Academy of Pediatrics recommends the first visit not later than 12 months. Many general dentists do not feel comfortable treating very young children, so some dentists may put off treating infants as a result.

Baby teeth serve several important functions. They help the jaws grow to their proper size and they hold space to guide the permanent teeth into their proper locations. If you were to lose the front four teeth (incisors) top and bottom, early, the loss will not have too much impact. For children over the age of two who lose a front baby tooth early, it is almost exclusively a cosmetic concern. Back molars lost to severe decay can potentially prevent the jaw from growing to its normal size. Removing the decayed tooth, even though it is "just a baby tooth" can be a huge mistake. If cavities do occur, it is important to repair them for three reasons: to avoid pain and toothaches, to chew with until your child is almost a teenager, and to prevent unnatural shifting of the teeth which can keep the jaw from attaining its normal size, cause orthodontic problems, and crowding.

The best dentistry is the least dentistry. Repairing any tooth is not ideal; any restoration is not going to be as durable as what nature created for us in the first place. It is very difficult to fix front baby teeth in an ideal manner. Most of the repair materials that look nice (white fillings) are not very sturdy, while the ones that are sturdy (stainless steel caps) don't look appealing. Dental problems are an infectious disease. A little cavity left untreated becomes a bigger cavity, then it becomes a toothache, and finally it becomes an abscess. Each time a dentist does a restoration, it weakens the tooth. When that repair "wears out" a new repair must be done. Each repair becomes larger and weakens the tooth a little more. A little gum disease (gingivitis) left untreated becomes bigger gum disease (periodontitis) -- a friend of mine, Dr. Michael Schuster, calls this "The Dreadful Story." *Avoiding fillings, caps and other repairs to the teeth through better overall health is the goal. If you can keep your child cavity-free until the teenage years, you might be able to keep him or her cavity-free for life. If you can keep your teenager from having gingivitis, you can prevent him or her from having gum disease as an adult.*

As we get older our decay rate generally drops. As we leave adolescence behind, our dental problems usually take two forms: We need to replace an old filling either because it has worn out or decay has occurred in the tiny gap between where the filling stops and the tooth starts, or we start to develop gum disease in the form of gingivitis (mild) or periodontitis (more severe). Most adults needing fillings are not filling new cavities – they are most often re-filling the cavities of their youth. Both the bacteria that cause cavities and those that cause gum disease produce inflammation in our body. This inflammation causes stress on our system and the production of something called "C-reactive proteins." Three things, which are directly related to dental disease – stress, inflammation, and C-reactive proteins, can be related to heart disease and diabetes. No one wants to increase their child's chances of any of those diseases. So those baby teeth aren't JUST baby teeth. As Dr. Mayo said, "If a person can take care of their teeth and gums they can extend their life by at least 10 years." We all want that for our children.

TEN WAYS TO ADD TEN YEARS TO YOUR CHILD'S LIFE:

1. **Cleaning their mouth** – The earlier you start oral hygiene care the better. Start cleaning your child's mouth the very first day. After feeding, clean the infant's mouth with damp gauze or a clean washcloth. This reduces the number of harmful bacteria in the mouth and allows healthy (probiotic) bacteria to survive. As soon as your child has a tooth you should be brushing it. To start a toothbrush with just water is fine. As your child grows, introduce an infant tooth and gum cleaner. When they are close to two years old, introducing them to toothpaste is fine. Toothpaste advertisements demonstrate a giant "S"-shaped glob of toothpaste. A child should use an amount of toothpaste equal to about the size of half a garden pea or just enough to color the bristles. Ingesting too much can cause fluorosis or staining

of the teeth. People who live in urban centers get flouride in their water. Additionally, some children may be taking a multivitamin with fluoride, or using a mouth rinse containing fluoride. If the child is using these products and they also swallow too much toothpaste, problems can occur. Parental supervision is the key. Floss as soon as there are two teeth in the mouth that touch each other. Until then, if there is space between teeth, a brush should reach those spaces. This will also help keep gum disease 'at bay' down the road. There are aids to make flossing in a child's mouth easier. Try those handy little flossers that look like crayons or dinosaurs. They are an easier and more fun way to get children to let mom and dad help them floss.

2. **First dental visit when their first tooth comes in or by 12 months of age** – An early check by your dentist can go a long way to preventing problems. Your dentist can also counsel you on how to best care for your child's teeth and point out problems when they are small and are easy to correct. If your dentist says that your child is too young and suggests waiting until they are bigger, do not take no for an answer. Find a pediatric dentist and schedule your child for an appointment (Find one at The American Academy of Pediatric Dentists website at: www. aadp.org). Every day in my office I see several children under the age of four with severe decay and infection. Don't let your child be one.

3. **Keep up their brushing and flossing** – Caregiver help. How long should you help them to brush and floss? Studies show that most children do not have

coordination to brush their own teeth until they are 8 years old. Many are even older before they can be responsible. Letting them brush unsupervised can result in about a 4 second brushing time. So it's okay to help your child brush and floss. If you have to bargain with them, some children wish to be independent, let them brush in the morning (supervised) then you brush for them before bed.

4. **Teething and discomfort** – Teething and teething remedies. There are lots of 'old wives' tales about treating tooth pain. One is to put aspirin or Tylenol directly onto the sore spot. If you have a headache you wouldn't tape two aspirin to your forehead! Medicine applied directly to the sore spot on teeth or gums can be acidic and can burn the gums. The best teething remedy is to use one of those liquid-filled, soft teething rings that you can chill in the refrigerator and get cool for them to chew on. Second best is an oral pain remedy like Tylenol or Motrin. Third best is Orajel or the like that are over the counter, topical pain relievers, but these remedies do have a tendency to dry out the gums. You just don't want to use them too many times a day.

5. **Toothpastes** –When a child is very young, a toothbrush with water is fine. For toddlers, an infant tooth and gum cleanser is best. For children over age 30 months, any of the toothpaste with the American Dental Association Seal of Acceptance is fine, just be careful to supervise and not let them swallow the toothpaste.

6. **Which Toothbrush?** – With all kids you should

use a soft bristle brush with end-rounded bristles. Medium and Hard brushes are just too hard on teeth and gums. Their brush should be replaced at least every 3 months or if the child has been ill. If they were sick, you should pitch the brush and get a new one. Make it fun – they will brush longer. A common question from parents is on the use of an electric toothbrush versus a manual toothbrush. I personally do not think that any one brush is better than another as far as brand or electric or manual. However, if the electric toothbrush will get them to brush longer, then that is the best choice. The recommended pediatric guideline is two minutes of brushing. Whatever time you can get them to sit still for brushing is better than no time. If you select an electric toothbrush, start out slowly. There are some great semi-disposable and inexpensive brands of toothbrushes that you can try with your child to establish if he or she likes the sensation of the electric toothbrush before you invest in one that is more expensive. There are also many novelty-type pediatric toothbrushes, such as those that play music that will get your child interested in brushing.

7. **Orthodontic Care** – Early Orthodontics. Most children should have their first visit with an orthodontist shortly after their first permanent teeth come in. Early consultation with an orthodontist can improve the final result and may even reduce treatment time and costs. If a child has moderate to severe crowding problems, early treatment by the orthodontist can help prevent removal of the permanent teeth that was so common

in orthodontic care in the 1960s and 1970s. In my practice I generally will send a child that I perceive to have moderate orthodontic problems between the ages of six and eight years. With severe problems where the child has "bulldog bite" or "Dick Tracy" jaw – in which the lower jaw sticks way out – I will send them earlier. Orthodontics is not just about cosmetics. Straighter teeth make it easier to prevent cavities and gum disease. Remember, while undergoing braces, your child still needs to see your family dentist or pediatric dentist.

8. **Good eating habits** – Good nutrition and eating habits go a long way to help keep your mouth and entire body healthy. There are many good books on this subject; take time to read a few. The thing to remember is for decay and gum disease to occur, three components must be present: teeth, bacteria, and sugars (carbohydrates). The bacteria really do not care what kind of sugar it is; they can work with any of them to cause disease. What you need to remember is the biggest factor is how often you are exposing your mouth to sugar. Sipping juice, soda, or milk all day long can be very rough on teeth.

9. **Regular Dental Care** – For most people this means an exam and cleaning every six months. This should be individualized for each person. If a child has a high decay rate, they may need to be seen more often. A child who has great oral hygiene and low decay rate may be seen less frequently.

10. **It's in your hands** – A dental professional can do a

great deal to help you and your child reach optimal oral health but it is really up to you, the parent. The dentist will probably see you 2 to 4 times a year. They are really your coach to help you get there. The other 360+ days you are the one taking care of their mouth. Ultimately, you will have the greatest impact on whether or not you are successful.

My goal as a pediatric dentist is to help families recognize that dental health is a major component of overall health. Those early teeth are "not just baby teeth." Primary teeth should be valued and cared for in the same way that you care for your child's ten fingers and toes. Early dental care can act like a vaccine to safeguard overall health. Can you think of any reason why you wouldn't wish to add ten years to your child's life?

ABOUT WILLIAM

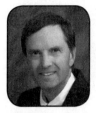

William (Bill) J. Donhiser, DDS is a pediatric dentist, entrepreneur, businessman and best selling author who wishes to help people enjoy good dental and overall health by avoiding the problems he has seen in many of his young patients.

Dr. Donhiser received his education from The University of Wyoming (B.S. with honors), The Medical College of Virginia (D.D.S.), Wright State University's Children Medical Center, and University of Indiana (Certificate in Pediatric Dentistry), and has completed the Executive Management Program at Kellogg School of Business, Northwestern University in Chicago.

He founded Black Hills Pediatric Dentistry in 1985, now a six-dentist specialty practice serving the dental needs of children in a five state area. Dr. Donhiser has been a founding member of two Licensed Specialty Hospitals and one Outpatient Surgical Center. He has served as Chairman of the Board of two of these facilities. Bill also is involved in real-estate development, having built two surgical centers, one professional office complex and two retail centers.

Currently Dr. Donhiser spends most of his professional time treating children with Early Childhoods Caries (cavities), who are unable to tolerate treatment in a dental office, in surgery centers under general anesthesia.

In his leisure time, Dr. Donhiser is a voracious reader and lifelong student. He enjoys active outdoor sports (snow skiing, hiking, bicycling) and traveling with his wife and three children.

CHAPTER 10

SECRETS TO A YOUNGER LOOKING FACE

BY ALLEN SMUDDE, DDS
& KELLY SMUDDE, DDS

Most people are looking for ways to look younger and healthier regardless of their age. In social settings, when we are first introduced, we immediately notice the other person's face. We look for signs of friendliness, confidence, intelligence, and health, and then we create an overall judgment of that person based on what we determine by our assessment of their look. What we see when we look at a person's face is merely the thin layer of skin that covers over their skeletal structure below. The jawbones and teeth make up most of the delicate support structure of any face that we see. If you lose your jawbones, your face will lose its form and appear to "cave in". Because of the lack of bone structure underneath, there will be less support for your skin, which causes voids that make your face appear wrinkled. The best way to prevent the appearance of aging in over half of the visible area on your face is to keep your underlying jawbone healthy and free of disease. There are two major ways to maintain the health of your jawbone. The first is prevention, and the second is dental implants.

Ben Franklin's famous quote, "An ounce of prevention is worth a pound of cure," definitely pertains to dentistry. The number one secret to a more youthful face is the prevention of bone loss through dental cleanings. Common sense tells us that we need to eat and to drink to sustain our lives, and that all foods and beverages must pass through your mouth in order to have the desired effect. Therefore, it follows that your teeth are going to need the constant and ongoing care and attention of a qualified dental team. By way of food and saliva, bacteria unavoidably get caught in and around your teeth. Brushing and flossing alone only cleanse the visible 1/3 of your tooth structure, leaving 2/3 of your teeth unattended. The only way to remove the tenacious deadly bacteria that form underneath your gums, above your gums, and around your teeth and bones is to get your teeth professionally cleaned at your dental office.

Why is having bacteria in your mouth so dangerous? Tooth enamel is the hardest structure in the human body. If these bacteria can so easily degrade the structure of the tooth, eat holes in your teeth, and cause cavities, just imagine what they can do to all of the body's more delicate structures. Many different strains of bacteria hide in the crevices of your mouth and destroy the structures around them. One example of this type of destruction is periodontal disease. Over 80% of the population will get periodontal disease at some point in their lives. Periodontal disease is a rapidly progressive, incurable disease whereby the bacteria in your mouth consume your jawbones. The bacteria are so tenacious that they are able to eat away your gums, then your jawbones, and eventually cause tooth loss. When you have lost both teeth and bone, you have lost the underlying support structure for the bulk of your face.

How often should you get your teeth professionally cleaned? This is a decision for you and your body to make along with the guidance of your dental team. Never rely on an extraneous source like an insurance company to dictate how frequently you have your teeth cleaned. As a guideline, we tell our patients to mark their calendars the day they have their cleaning and then to look for plaque formation around their lower front teeth. The day they see bacteria accumulate in the form of plaque is the day they should return for their next cleaning. If your teeth need a cleaning every three months, but you choose to go every six months, this neglect could result in incurable bone loss. Remember, bone is the structure that holds your face in place.

In a related situation, why does the guy sitting next to me on the airplane always seem to have bad breath? I know it sounds funny, but patients ask questions like this quite often. If you always want to assure that you have good breath, one way is to practice a few dental prevention techniques. The most important technique is to get thorough and comprehensive cleanings. When you miss dental cleanings, bacteria build up and accumulate. Those same bacteria then consume your gingivae (your gums) and bones; at which point your breath starts to smell like rotting flesh.

Bad breath is one of the indicators of periodontal disease. The longer periodontal disease is left untreated, the more jawbone the disease will consume. Teeth that are cleaned often will project both good health and youthfulness.

Dental implants are dentistry's secret weapon against a prematurely aging face. When tooth loss occurs, the surrounding bone structure melts away. When you lose teeth, your body's natural physiologic response is to determine that the bone that was holding the tooth in place now represents an unnecessary expenditure of its energy to maintain. That is to say that the body interprets your jaw as no longer being useful to your teeth to chew, and therefore the bone mass of your jaw gets reabsorbed back into the body. The more consecutive teeth that are lost (teeth next to each other), the more noticeably the bone erodes. When a person loses all of their teeth, the jawbones eventually disintegrate so much that they become barely visible on an x-ray. As a person loses most of the bone support of their jaw, their face collapses inward and they lose the vertical dimension of their facial appearance. This makes wearing a denture or a removable partial appliance uncomfortable, if not almost impossible, since there is nothing solid (in the form of bone) to hold it in place.

Patients who have lost all of their lower teeth are at an increased susceptibility to jaw fractures as well, due to their lack of bone support and torque forces while chewing. Also, if the jawbone is allowed to disintegrate naturally after tooth loss, the bony encasement that protects the jaw's nerves eventually erodes and becomes exposed which causes severe pain to patients. Chewing, and even putting on a denture, becomes a painful undertaking. Aging gracefully by allowing all of your teeth to fall out is a less palatable option for those who are concerned with maintaining their health and cosmetic appearance well into their mature years.

Are dental implants the only option for missing teeth? No. You can have a fixed bridge placed or a removable denture fabricated for you. Both serve to fill in the gaps that previously housed the teeth in the mouth. Secondly, both options help to prevent the adjacent teeth from misaligning and causing numerous future problems. Thirdly, both bridges and dentures prevent the super-eruption of the teeth in the opposite jaw. That is to say, when a tooth is missing, and teeth in the opposite jaw do not have an occlusal match, they erupt until they eventually hit the opposite gingivae (gum), thus causing future dental problems. Bridges and dentures do **not** preserve the jawbones and prevent bone deterioration where the tooth is missing. The most comprehensive solution to maintain the integrity of your teeth, keep your gums healthy and preserve the underlying jawbone is still dental implants.

Now that we know that they are the best solution for replacing missing teeth, we should now properly define just what exactly **is** a dental implant? A dental implant is a titanium fixture that is gently placed into the jawbone where the natural tooth root once was. There are three parts to an implant. The titanium implant body is placed first. Once this implant body is placed, it requires several months to fuse with the jaw around it and become part of your bone. During this time, a temporary crown may be made for aesthetic purposes. Secondly, the implant abutment is the component that fits on top of and screws into the implant body. Thirdly, the implant crown is fabricated to naturally emanate over the abutment and into the smile line. The implant crown is the only portion of the implant that is outwardly visible to you and to others. It looks like a natural tooth. Having gotten to this point, it's only natural to wonder if the implants are painful when placed in your mouth. Good news! Patients report feeling minimal discomfort. This is mainly because the area of the bone where the implant is placed does not have nerves. Implant placement is an outpatient surgery that can be done under local anesthetic. The procedure usually takes less than an hour or two depending upon the individual's surgical needs.

So an implant is the best way to go if prevention fails, and they don't hurt when they're placed in the mouth, but how long do they last? Good question! The success rate thus far is about 95% within the 50 years that clinical research has been done on implants. This is a much greater success rate than dental crowns and bridges can boast. The reason for this is that dentures have to be remade because the supporting jawbone underneath them deteriorates and alters the fit.

Similarly, bridges rely on at least three teeth to maintain, so there are greater odds of failure there. Of course, the outstanding success rate of your implants depends partially on you, and how you care for them. Fortunately they are brushed and flossed just like your natural teeth. Your dental professional will use special instruments to clean each individual implant during your cleanings. X-rays will be taken to continually evaluate your bone health underneath. Surgical implants are now a part of your body, and therefore will be just as susceptible to periodontal disease as your natural teeth are, so proper cleanings are important for good health.

Now, are implants the right choice for everyone? Not everyone. Though most people are candidates for implants, children and young adults whose bones are still growing will need to defer treatment until those bones have fully developed. Also, certain medical complications may limit treatment. A consultation with your dentist and surgeon will allow a more thorough evaluation of your needs.

In conclusion, good preventive dentistry is by far, the easiest way to maintain your youthful facial appearance. By preserving your teeth, you're also preserving your smile, and you're projecting good health to all those in your company. Once a tooth is lost, immediately replacing it with an implant will preserve the underlying bone structure that makes up your face for years to come. With the prevention of dental diseases and the preservation of the structures that make up your face, dentistry really is so much "More than a Mouthful."

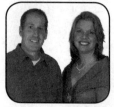

ABOUT ALLEN AND KELLY

Drs. Allen and Kelly Smudde are a husband and wife team practicing in Valencia, CA. They were both born in Indiana, and met in Chicago at Northwestern University. Allen moved from Terre Haute, IN to La Canada, CA when he was 10 years old, and Kelly grew up on a farm in Valparaiso, IN. It was not until they were at their wedding reception on Dr. Kelly's farm in Indiana that they realized that both of their fathers had a mutual roommate while at Indiana University Dental School, and all were reunited at their wedding. They both come from a long line of dentists in the family. Allen's father and several family members are dentists, and Kelly is a fourth generation dentist. They both started learning dentistry from their earliest memories onward and both spent many hours in their parents' labs hand-sculpting teeth out of wax and hand-making jewelry.

They are continually building upon the foundation of skills that they learned as children – so that they can provide you and your family with the best that dentistry has to offer.

Education:

Dr. Kelly Smudde attended Culver Military Academy for eight summers. Her family has attended Culver for over 70 years. Dr. Kelly attended Saint Mary's College in Notre Dame, IN and is a Fighting Irish Fan. She then went on to attend Northwestern University School of Dentistry in Chicago. She did her residency at UCLA Sepulveda VA in LA.

Dr. Allen Smudde attended Flintridge Prep for high school in La Canada, CA, then Glendale Community College, and Humboldt State University in California. He then went on to attend Northwestern University School of Dentistry in Chicago. Dr. Allen did his residency at Northwestern Memorial Hospital VA in Chicago. (He likes the Fighting Irish too, ...along with The Northwestern Wildcats!)

Drs. Allen and Kelly Smudde can be reached at:

YourValenciaDentist.com, or by calling 661-259-4474.

They are located at: 27450 Tourney Road, Suite 250, Valencia, CA 91355.

CHAPTER 11

THE VITAL IMPORTANCE OF REPLACING MISSING TEETH

BY THOMAS M. KACHOREK, DDS

This book just might move you to take better care of your teeth, which in turn, could vastly improve or even save your life! Most people probably know very little about their teeth and how it affects their health, and more importantly- neither do many people in the health care industry. However, doctors industry-wide are beginning to understand that those people who get their teeth fixed and keep them healthy live longer, better quality lives. Some estimate this increase in longevity at ten years!

Healthy teeth help you function normally, help you effectively chew the foods you like to eat. They enable you to speak, smile and get along in life. They powerfully and directly affect your health. We know that your oral health has a direct relationship to the rest of your body. It affects your cardiovascular system, it affects arthritis, heart disease, stroke and diabetes too!

We're finding that the inflammation caused by the infections in your mouth, even the kind that doesn't hurt and remains invisible, affects your body's ability to handle stress in general.

Research is now pointing to inflammation as a probable cause of Alzheimer's disease. This horrible, debilitating condition chokes the life out of its victims and worsens the lives of caregivers, usually the family members who love them. Chronic, often symptom-less dental infections that so many older people have can and do, cause inflammation throughout the body. Many dental problems that numerous people have deemed "innocent" and "no big deal" could be a very big deal in what are supposed to be the golden years of life. Who wants to become a burden to their beloved ones? We already know that infections in the mouth can seep into the body from neglected and painless dental disease. Why put your future at risk unnecessarily?

YOU WILL NEED YOUR TEETH LONGER

Longevity is increasing. Today, we know that half of those who are age 60 or older are going to live to be in their nineties. We've made sweeping changes in how long people live. At the time that social security was implemented, the average life span was 47 years! So it was very easy to provide a system that gave retirement benefits at age 65.

Today, we're tipping out over 80 on average and it's climbing. With the Human Genome Project and the advances in nanotechnology, we expect that life spans are going to be over 100 years in the not-so-distant future.

One of the big lessons of this book is how to keep your teeth for your lifetime, even to age 100! *We want readers to not only add years to their life, but life to their years.*

The stories of patients told herein are of *real* patients. We have altered names and put these together to help you understand dental care and its benefits in a new way. The reality is that the new, more modern dentist can be a real source of greater health, a better quality of life and a longer one. The power they wield can be regenerative, even transformative to a whole new, better level of living.

Systemic problems can affect your dental health also. GERD, also known as Gastro Esophogeal Reflux Disease can breakdown the teeth rapidly, increase decay and cause a tooth-loss epidemic. All manners of systemic conditions and medications (over 400 to date) can cause dry mouth, alter the immune capabilities of the mouth and worsen gum disease and the ability to heal. Diabetes is among the worst culprits, increasing gum disease and tooth decay.

SMILING AS WE GROW OLDER

As we grow older our faces change. Gravity takes over. Between age 30 and age 70, we all experience significant facial changes that occur naturally because of gravity.

As we age, we get wrinkles. Our face starts to show the crow's feet at the eyes and laugh lines around our faces. We get brown spots. Often those who've had teeth removed but not sufficiently replaced, get more wrinkles. They look older – far older than their natural age. The changes in diet due to impaired or altered chewing ability further advance the aging process, often making one look 10 to 20 years older than actual age.

Often people start to loose their back teeth and think it's OK. There are no symptoms – yet. As you loose more of your molar teeth, it means you have to chew on your front teeth. Front teeth were not designed for grinding, but for shearing food – like a pair of scissors. So trying to grind on your front teeth wears them out much faster and can completely change your smile.

THE SMILE – DOMINANT FACE

The good news comes from the "smile-dominant" face. It consists of a smile that is so big and bright and beautiful that the facial wrinkles and blemishes fade into insignificance. This smile-dominant faces look younger, healthier and more vibrant. A patient of mine recently said, "It's better and easier than plastic surgery."

On the other hand, if you're one of those people that hide their smile (the opposite of a smile-dominant face) people see and focus on those wrinkles, blemishes, lines and spots. Wouldn't you rather have a gorgeous smile that people focus on instead?

LIVING LONGER, LIVING BETTER

As we said earlier, people are living longer. So we need our teeth longer, right? You probably don't think about it, but how you look and interact with your children and grandchildren is part of the real legacy that you leave for them. Part of your legacy is how the people you love and who love you, remember you.

Quite frankly, your smile can help you leave a legacy of cheer, love and joy. When your family thinks of you, they can think of you as having that great gorgeous smile and a happy demeanor. That legacy can be a difference-maker far into the future.

WORN OUT DENTISTRY

A lot of folks in the boomer age group, all 78 million of them, have old dentistry that has worn out. If you have dental work that is 15, 20, 25 years old, you are going to need to have more work done. This happens to everyone, it's just a matter of time. Old, dark, stained and worn fillings will need replacement. Leaving failing dentistry in place threatens the health of the teeth by increasing the likelihood of decay and infection into the nerve within the tooth. You should check with your dentist to see when the right time is to replace old dentistry. Being proactive on this will help prevent future pain and increased expense.

Boomers don't want to sit on a porch in a rocking chair, chomping their dentures together. Healthy teeth can play a major role in giving you that quality and quantity of living that you'd like to have. If you can't eat right, the quality of your life diminishes along with your health. Besides, eating what you want comfortably is one of life's true pleasures, wouldn't you agree?

REBECCA'S STORY

For Rebecca, losing her teeth and getting dentures at age 52 had been an unhappy choice she confided in us.

"At the time, I thought it was the least worse decision I could make. I had had trouble with my teeth for my entire life. I was glad to be rid of them. It was true that I had to focus a lot of attention on my false teeth. I couldn't eat what I wanted all the time. And after being re-fitted with new ones, my chewing was easier, but it wasn't long until my bones had shrunk more, and once again I experienced insecurity about being out in public. I really hated that. It felt so confining."

"I had heard about dental implants, but thought they were going to be too expensive, so I just tried to get along with my dentures."

"One weekend, I was keeping my little treasure, my three year old granddaughter, Brittany. Sometimes blessings come from unusual places. She watched me putting in my dentures. I could see her eyes get big. She said "Granny, why do you have teeth that you put in?" I was crushed. I didn't want this little light of my life thinking about me in any way like that. Plus, I knew I wasn't eating like I should. That's when I decided to call you."

After an examination and complete dental physical, we came up with a plan for Rebecca. We placed dental implants and made teeth for her that didn't come out. Rebecca loves her new smile and the comfort of knowing she wouldn't have any embarrassing denture moments ever again.

We know what Rebecca wanted even if she couldn't, wouldn't and didn't know how to say what it was.

"When I am gone, I want her and all my grandchildren to remember me as the loving, smiling, kind grandmother – not as the unsmiling woman who took her teeth in and out."

"I am so-o-o-o glad I had this done and I feel better about me. I feel more energized than before. And I am enjoying my food better than I have in years."

REMOVABLE TEETH – DENTURES AND PARTIAL DENTURES

Man is the only animal that can continue living without its teeth. Take the teeth away from any other animal and it dies.

Take the teeth away from man and there are choices. For some, removable teeth are the only solution. Others choose the better, more permanent solution afforded by today's technology – implants!

In many respects, dentures are like oral wigs. Like a toupée or wig, they are but pale versions of the original, and most don't look very good.

Dentures are like that, too. They sit on top of your gums. *Some* can look pretty good. Many don't.

But because they're sitting on top of your gums, the force of chewing goes through the dentures to the soft tissue and bone underneath. Frequently, the soft tissue under a full or partial denture develops painful sore spots. The compression on the bone caused by the chewing on dentures inevitably leads to loss of bone. It is but a matter of time.

This loss of bone occurs in both height and width. This bone loss of the upper and lower jaws over time leads to wrinkles, and for many, facial disfigurement.

Bone loss itself makes dentures more difficult to wear over time. There is just less to hold onto. I feel very sorry for the people in their 60's, 70's or 80's, who see dentures as the only solution to their problem. Why? Because their ability to accommodate new dentures is decreased just because of their age. As we grow older, our ability to accommodate dentures decreases as we grow older.

Many dentures are made slap-dash for economic reasons. These poorly fitting dentures worsen bone loss all by themselves. This loss of bone further worsens the fit which further worsens the bone loss. This continues in a dwindling spiral with the denture wearer the biggest loser.

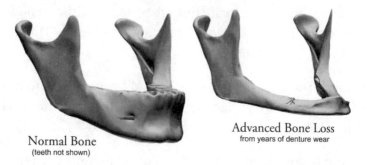

Normal Bone
(teeth not shown)

Advanced Bone Loss
from years of denture wear

The average denture wearer should have his denture relined or remade within one year of first receiving them. After three years, another reline is probably necessary. After seven years, a new set is needed. Few denture wearers adhere to a schedule of care like this at all. In fact, the average denture wearer goes to a dentist once every 14.9 years! There is a huge gap between what should be and what the public typically does. This failure to see a need for care makes the denture experience worse and puts the denture wearer at risk for increased oral cancer, especially for smokers.

DENTURE ADHESIVES

Denture adhesives have been around a long time. These are used to help stabilize dentures. In the U.S. alone, over 200 million dollars a year is spent buying the material. Evidently a lot of people want removable teeth that don't move around!

The poorer the fit of the dentures, the greater the use of the 'goop' to hold them in place. The poorer the fit, the greater the bone loss caused by the ill-fitting dentures! The very thing that is supposed to be helping is causing more loss of bone!

Is there ever a good use for a denture adhesive? Yes, there is. When a person wants the extra security that the adhesive gives them in public places, an adhesive can help out. No one wants to see a person's teeth fall out onto the plate in a restaurant. The real question is how much should be used? Just a tiny smidgen spread out over the whole denture. That is all that it should take to ratchet up the adherence to the tissues. It is so little that it is barely visible.

If the denture wearer is requiring more that just a little, then the likelihood is that the dentures should be replaced with better fitting ones.

WHAT ABOUT PARTIAL DENTURES?

Given the choice between having no teeth or wearing a full denture, the partial denture can be a better choice. Why? Because a well-made partial denture distributes the bite force onto the remaining teeth as much as possible, away from the bone. This requires the partial denture to be rigid, usually made of metal and specifically made to use the teeth as anchors and retention of the partial denture. However, just like the full denture, the gum and bone underneath the partial recede in time.

Here is a real surprise: 40% of partial dentures stay in drawers, worn not at all or just for special occasions. Frequently, a person can chew better without the partial denture!

Creating a well-made partial denture is a tall order. Even when done well, many people find partials too uncomfortable to wear. Many people consider the hooks of the partial denture fitting onto the remaining teeth to be so unsightly that they refuse to wear them.

Statistically speaking, teeth that anchor partial dentures are more likely to decay or get loose from the force put against them by the partial. If you are saying to yourself, "Why would anyone want a partial denture?" I understand. They should be avoided if possible.

WHAT TO DO IF YOU ARE LOSING YOUR TEETH

Removable teeth are generally a poor solution for everyone. Avoid them if you can. If you must lose your teeth consider how you could keep some tooth roots. Saving two to four roots will help maintain your bone levels and help hold your denture in place. Dentures that fit over tooth roots are called overdentures, meaning that the dentures fit over the roots and come in and out just like regular dentures do. But the difference is we can get the overdenture to "snap" into place on your roots, keeping them in your mouth nice and tight. Overdentures are a real God-send when dental implants don't fit into a person's budget.

WHAT TO DO IF YOU ALREADY HAVE DENTURES

For many people, dentures were the only option they had in the past when they lost their teeth. The reason, no matter what it was then, is now removed. Today you no longer have to wear dentures. The best option is to have dental implant treatment that protects and stimulates the bone to remain. This generally requires a number of implants sufficient to support the replacement teeth. Interestingly, the number of implants needed is dependent on a person's age, bite function, total body size, density of bone and total bone volume. Everyone is different so there is no standard number to use. The number, type and size of dental implants is based on diagnoses of your individual needs.

DENTURE REALITY

The more effort, expertise and talent that are brought to bear in making dentures, the better the fit, longevity and success of denture service. It is no surprise when economy dentures fail. True, a few people can tolerate anything, but they are the rare exceptions, only a few out of a thousand patients can muster the energy to make quickie dentures really work – to tolerate them in spite of all the problems. Many a patient has been severely disappointed to learn about the inadequacies of these kinds of dentures thorough first-hand experience.

Making a set of dentures that are custom-fit to match your level of bone, facial appearance, muscles, tongue and jaw movements is the best denture service investment.

One problem we commonly see is "clacking" dentures. It's embarrassing. They make noise all the time. Generally, that indicates one of two things. The dentures are either too close together, or there's so little bone that the muscles in the floor of the mouth force the dentures up – making that clacking sound as the teeth of the upper and lower denture come together.

FINAL RECOMMENDATIONS

- If you must have dentures, get the best ones possible from an experienced dentist that makes high quality dentures on a regular basis. The dentist should make customize impressions, tooth arrangement and match the color of your gums.
- Replace your dentures every 7-8 years.
- Get relines every 2-4 years as needed to keep your dentures fitting as well as possible.
- Let your mouth rest at least 4 hours a day by removing your denture.

If it is possible for you, get dental implants to avoid becoming toothless. If you are already a denture wearer, find a way to get dental implants. They can change your life.

As much as I've told you about dentures, understand this: anytime that you can use dental implants or natural teeth in a healthy mouth instead of removable teeth, you're better off.

For some people, dentures are the only solution. In that case, get them made as well as you possibly can. But if possible, choose the alternative, dental implants.

What if my jaws have shrunk so much that I can't get implants, or, I just want to make my dentures from slipping out all the time?

Good news! We have something new that helped thousands of patients. As a matter of fact, it's the biggest growing thing we do. "Mini-implants!" These are very thin pegs that go into the jaw without cutting, without sutures and without pain! They look like little screws and they hold the denture in place – but good. Yes, without adhesives, without getting food underneath them. You can chew much harder with confidence. You can bite into an apple, eat ribs, salad, steak – all without coming loose. You can smile, talk, kiss, laugh, cough and sneeze – knowing they'll stay in place!

The whole procedure takes less than two hours and there is virtually no pain afterwards. Once these mini-implants are in, they help prevent the jaws from shrinking any further. These mini-implants also will fit comfortably into people's budgets!

On occasion, I do come across some people that have almost no bone left to do these procedures. They tell me they would pay a million dollars to have their procedure done just so they could eat and get nutrition, because they are literally dying. They told me to *promise* to tell everyone without teeth, that they should get either the implants or mini-implants before it is too late! Unfortunately, that time comes more rapidly than we think.

So, I am doing what I promised. I want everyone to know to try to save their teeth for life. And if you don't have teeth, talk to a dentist as soon as possible for an evaluation to see if you can get implants, or at least mini-implants. It could save your life! Not to mention you'll be able to eat, get proper nutrition, look 10 years younger, smile, and talk with confidence. Leave your legacy, live your life, be happy and healthy! I've done my part, now for health's sake – do yours.

LORI'S STORY

Losing a tooth here and there hadn't seemed a big deal for Lori.

"They were in the back. No one could really see they were missing. Or so I thought. It was at my niece's wedding reception that I heard the comment that shook me awake. I'll never forget it, 'Kim's Aunt Lori looks so old compared to Kim's mom. Those missing teeth would make you think she is from the backwoods, a hillbilly or something.'"

"It was one of those bathroom conversations that were supposed to be private. I happened to be in there freshening up at the same time. I ran out with tears welling up in my eyes. I tried to forget about it and put on my social face. I couldn't stop thinking about those words. I excused myself and went to find a mirror where I could look at my face and smile privately. I found one and I took a good look. I didn't like what I saw. I wondered how many other people were saying to themselves what that young hussy had said!"

"I am five years younger than Kim's mom, my sister, Lindsey. She looks like early 40's, late 30's!"

"I started thinking about it, comparing Lindsey's smile to mine. I realized that I didn't look 50, I looked more like 60. My face had more wrinkles. My smile was dark, teeth were twisted and uneven. The mirror set I had found let me view my smile from the side. That's when I realized how much all those missing teeth showed and all the missing support for my face."

Lindsey sent Lori to us. We were able to get her smile rejuvenation done by using dental implants, smile design and some newer therapies to regain lost bone. You should see her smile now. Lori later told us, "It was a significant investment and it took more time and money that I thought it would. And I wish I had done something years ago. After you explained about my gum disease, I know this wasn't just about my looks; it was about my health, too. I feel better now than I have in twenty years."

Lori had a nasty case of gum disease that would have caused her to lose all her teeth had she delayed treatment any longer. Plus with what we now know about the mouth-body interactions and her family history of heart disease and cancer, Lori's decision to get her smile back and teeth healthy again might just have saved her life. It was about three months after we had completed her extensive makeover with dental implants, that we saw Lori again for her now regular maintenance visit. The ring on her finger said it all. After being divorced for five years, she now had found the new love of her life. She smiled. She was beaming.

"Other people need to know about this. Most people don't know how important your smile and oral health is to your happiness and health," Lori says.

We agree. That is one of the reasons for this book.

ABOUT THOMAS

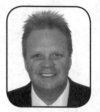

Dr. Thomas Kachorek is part of a Clinton Township tradition of dental comfort and care. He is a 1983 graduate of the University of Detroit School of Dentistry, and has dedicated his professional career to providing you with the best that dentistry has to offer. Dr. Kachorek is continually educating himself and his staff on the newest dental techniques in order to provide his patients with advanced, state-of-the-art, comfortable, personalized, trusted and antiseptic dental care.

Dr. Kachorek has completed over 1,500 hours of continuing education courses in general and cosmetic dentistry. In the last 28 years, he has studied with many cosmetic and implant dentists and is currently working on his Master's in the Academy of General Dentistry. He was voted one of America's top dentists by the Consumers Research Council of America in Washington, D.C. He was also honored to be included in HOUR Detroit magazine for being selected by a vote of his peers as a "Top Dentist" for the last four years in a row.

Dr Kachorek has himself lectured extensively and has coached other dentists throughout the U.S. He has served on the board of the University of Detroit's Continuing Education Committee. He is currently a member of the American Dental Association, Michigan Dental Association, Macomb Dental Society, Academy of Cosmetic Dentistry, and a Fourth Degree member in the Knights of Columbus.

Dr. Kachorek authored a consumers guide to dentistry book entitled, "Say Cheese," in 2010. He gives talks throughout the Metro Detroit area on general health and diabetes.

He currently has a private practice in Clinton Township, Michigan. If you have any questions about dental treatment and diabetes, or about dentures, implants, etc., please look up his practice on line at: www.BaypointeDental.com or call (586) 263-1241. Either way, they will make sure to answer your questions and send information to you.

CHAPTER 12

MAKING EVERY SMILE COUNT

BY ZAN BEAVER, DMD

In searching for ideas for this book, I began asking friends and family " What are some topics of interest to people about their smile?" The typical response I received was " Just that question sounds boring". " Don't over think it and be so doctor- like". Tell people the 3 most important things they need to know to keep their teeth and gums healthy for a lifetime". So I spent months thinking about it. Everyone loves to talk about how cosmetic dentistry changed their life at parties and social gatherings. While the cosmetic imaging, amazing materials and advanced techniques available in todays cosmetic dental practice are very sexy, it only applies to a small portion of the general public. Not everyone is interested in a Hollywood smile. Some people just want to keep their teeth for a lifetime or replace certain teeth to enjoy the foods they love or just speak properly. So I decided to make available simple information that anyone could use to immediately improve the quality of their life with little effort and a small commitment to their health and self-esteem. It all boils down to a manageable readers digest version that anyone can understand and immediately adopt to maximize their oral health. Drum roll please...... Brush, floss, and visit your dentist regularly. Thanks for reading this enlightening material and that's all you need to know – just kidding.

Brushing is the first key. Most people who make their way into my practice are already brushing their teeth. They just need a little coaching on their technique. I recommend a soft bristle toothbrush, never hard, and the use of an American Dental Association approved fluoride toothpaste. You should be brushing twice a day at minimum. If you are averse to Fluoride, Tom's –All Natural Toothpaste is a good alternative. Electric toothbrushes are fantastic but not a necessity. You really don't have to use toothpaste at all to effectively clean your teeth.

Flossing, on the other hand , is the dark horse of dental hygiene. As a dentist, it is one the hardest things I do to try to convince people to floss daily. Everybody seems to know they need to floss but nobody wants the floss lecture. Every time I floss I am reminded that I don't particularly enjoy any aspect of this tedious hygiene measure. It is messy, inconvenient and more often than not – Gross. I cannot tell you how many times I have been lying in bed at night just about to drift off to sleep when I realize I did not floss my teeth. Skipped it in the normal routine for some reason - again. So, because I am a dentist and feel not only a personal obligation but professional one as well, I drag myself into bathroom and tear off that wretched piece of string. You see, as much as I dislike this laborious task, I've got this floss monkey on my back, and it's good. I know too much, and hopefully, the information I am about to share with you will put a floss monkey squarely on your back as well.

Poor gum health, like gingivitis and periodontitis, has been linked to all sorts of other diseases and problems in other areas of the body. Research has shown heart attack, stroke, low birth weight, pre-term babies, respiratory diseases, pancreatic cancer and diabetes are all linked to gum disease. Like medicine, dental science is rapidly expanding in the areas of periodontology, oral surgery, implantology, endodontics and oral medicine. With this quantum leap forward, it has become more necessary for general dentist to work as a team with other dental specialist and the patients' physician in order to maximize the success of dental treatment. The general dentist in today's healthcare environment is finding it increasingly difficult to be "all things to all men" and do it all with excellence. Most general dentist today naturally gravitate towards the areas of dentistry they enjoy and can perform with a high level of skill. A solo practitioner will need the help of other doctors in order to provide the most favorable outcomes. With that being said, I do feel there is a major paradigm shift being made in the way people view their oral health as a thumbnail sketch of the body's overall health. As science continues to prove with each passing day the mouth truly is the gateway of health for the rest of the body.

Surprisingly, the most common chronic inflammatory condition people have is gum disease. When it is generalized throughout the mouth it is an infection about the size of the palm of your hand. The problem is it does not hurt most of the time. If a person is not visiting their dentist regularly they could walk around for years with this large infection and never know it. As periodontal disease progresses a person might notice there gums are sore, swollen, red or bleeding. They probably will have chronic bad breath as well.

So how do unhealthy gums cause damage to other parts of your body? As you develop plaque around the teeth it causes inflammation. Some people who are affected will notice they bleed when they brush or floss. If this is left untreated, gingivitis, the reversible form of the disease, can progress to periodontitis. This involves the loss of bone and tissue attachment, and eventually the teeth can become loose and fall out. If you don't treat the disease you can have bacteria enter the bloodstream and cause inflammation in other areas of the body. This inflammation occurs in the blood vessels which increases the chance of heart disease by two fold and stroke by three fold if left untreated.

Studies have shown that people with severe gum disease following the initial gum therapy, technically called scaling and root planning, showed a spike in the levels of factors associated with inflammation such as c-reactive protein. However, shortly after the completion of intensive gum therapy, the levels come down possibly dipping below original levels due to therapy. What that means to you is if you have gum disease and you brush, floss, or eat things that make your gums bleed, you can have a spike in these inflammatory markers in the blood stream. It is very important to get it treated as early in the process as possible. The study demonstrated that following intensive gum therapy and the placement of a local antibiotic, the inflammatory factors were significantly reduced. This in turn improves endothelial function or the ability of the cells that line your blood vessels to be healthier.

So what are the recommendations for gum health evaluation and therapy? Both for people that have no history of gum disease and those who have had a heart attack or have been diagnosed with heart disease, the American Dental Association recommends everyone **BRUSH** their teeth at least two times a day and **FLOSS** at least once a day. This is the recommendation to maintain good oral health. Unfortunately, many people don't even recognize they have periodontal disease because the signs and symptoms can be silent or not seen. This is particularly true for smokers who are at the greatest risk because many times they do not see the bleeding gums that are more readily seen in non-smokers. Smokers have an even greater need to see a dental professional for an evaluation. I see the day when a person who has been diagnosed with heart disease or has suffered a stroke will be seen by a dentist for a periodontal examination and care as a portion of their cardiac care.

The third simple key to keeping your teeth and gums healthy for a lifetime is visiting the dentist at least twice a year, maybe more often if you have history of gum disease. Every decision you make has a cost benefit ratio. In other words, is the cost of something worth the benefit or reward? Your brain makes thousands of these calculations everyday on a conscious and subconscious level. Choosing to make the commitment to floss daily or see your dentist regularly is no different than any of these other daily decisions. The mental gymnastics people perform when trying to make this decision can be quite comical. You would not believe some of the excuses I have heard from people explaining why they are unable to make their dental appointment. Here are just a few.

1. My car ran out of gas and I can't get to the gas station
2. I was pushing my car to the gas station and I developed a stomach Hernia – I'm on the way to the hospital right now.
3. I lost my car keys.
4. The city is paving my street and I can't get out of the driveway.
5. There are two wild Rottweilers outside the door to my apartment and I can't get out.

What are the barriers for people who know they need to make this commitment to the health of their smile? After attending countless seminars and reading hundreds of books written by dental experts, the general consensus is not enough time and money. In my experience, this is not completely accurate. When you need or want something, finding the time or money is a relatively small obstacle when compared to fear. Fear is what keeps the lion's share of people who do not visit the dentist regularly from doing what they know they need to do. Time and money barriers can be logically overcome through creative financing and convenience scheduling. Fear is not logical. Thankfully, through advancement in the area of sedation dentistry many of these people are finding their way back into the dental office and receiving the care they so desperately need. The secret to overcoming dental anxiety is finding a dental office that you like and trust 100%. This would include everyone in that office from the front desk, to the hygienist, dental assistants and doctors. Trust, care, concern and competence are all necessary ingredients in the recipe for a stress free dental visit.

It is my sincere desire that you are now empowered to follow through on a decision to respect yourself on a whole new level. Taking action on these three simple keys will go a long way in your quest to keep your teeth and gums healthy for a lifetime. If you have cosmetic concerns there are many options for improving the appearance of your smile and self image. This is what I have committed my life's work to be. In closing, I would like to share the story of my decision to choose dentistry as a profession. While a student at the University of North Carolina at Chapel, I was a varsity Cheerleader. On a Friday afternoon practicing circus stunts, one of our young ladies broke my front tooth – Cheerleading can be a pretty rough sport. The physical pain was moderate, but the psychological pain cut much deeper. Let me explain. It was Friday afternoon and I had a 7 pm flight to Jacksonville, Florida to meet my new girlfriend's parents – Our first meeting. My girlfriend (now my wife) had arranged for me to meet her best friends and attend a large party of her high school classmates. I would not consider myself vain, but I was extremely self-conscious to say the least and tried not to smile the whole weekend, covering my mouth with my hand when I laughed – it was a pretty miserable existence for that weekend. I can really understand how the appearance of your teeth can boost or destroy your self confidence, especially as a young person. I was able to see a dentist on Monday morning after my trip to Florida. He was able to restore my tooth in about an hour and I thought it was pure magic. He not only restored my tooth, he restored my soul in a way. It was on this day I fell in love with dentistry. Not just the technical aspect but what it can do to restore a person's spirit. It was on this day I committed my life to **Making Every Smile Count**.

ABOUT ZAN

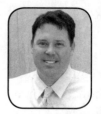

Dr. Beaver is passionate about teaching others inside and outside of his practice. He is an avid reader, writer and facebook enthusiast (www.facebook.com/beaverdental). He utilizes his extensive training and experience to treat even the most challenging dental situations. His commitment to "doing it right" and ability to "handle just about anything" through a dental team approach has won him the admiration of patients and other doctors. A big bonus is that Dr. Beaver uses his expertise to prevent big problems from ever happening.

Dr. Beaver graduated with honors from the University of North Carolina at Chapel Hill in 1995 and the University of Florida College of Dentistry in 1999. He has a long history of achievement from his younger days in high school, college and now in his professional life. Along the way he participated in football, track and played guitar in a band. As a senior in high school, he was captain of the football team and vice president of the student council.

As a collegian, he was a varsity cheerleader on a team that placed second in national competition. He worked as an ER technician at UNC hospitals emergency department to help pay for college and credits his love for medical and dental sciences to this experience.

In dental school, Dr. Beaver received numerous awards including the Omicron Kappa Upsilon Student Ethics Award, The Dentistry College Council's Student of the Year Award and the C.W. Fain Award for professionalism while a student at the University of Florida College of Dentistry. He was honored to be elected three consecutive years to serve on the Student Performance Evaluation Committee with faculty at the University of Florida College of Dentistry.

Dr. Beaver continued his education following graduation from dental school at the world renowned Dawson Center for Advanced Dental Studies and furthered his understanding of the art and science of dentistry with Dr. William Strupp, a nationally recognized pioneer in modern cosmetic dentistry. He is currently a member of the American Academy of Cosmetic Dentistry, the American Academy of Craniofacial Pain and the American Academy of Dental Sleep Medicine.

He has been helping patients so they can enjoy eating and smiling again with dental implants since 1999. Using a systematic team approach, Dr. Beaver can develop various options based on an individual's needs and budget while offering them a variety of solutions. He can help simplify even the most debilitated situations and often "rescue" the denture patient. In addition to cosmetics and implant dentistry he has a special interest in treating sleep apnea and utilizes one of the most comprehensive systems for treating tmj/ migraine sufferers available anywhere in the United States. He uses the most safe and predictable methods for oral conscious sedation to treat patients with high dental anxiety.

To learn more about Dr. Zan Beaver and how you can receive free special reports and other valuable information about the miracles of modern dentistry visit WWW.BeaverDental.com or Call 904-396-GRIN.

CHAPTER 13

DEALING WITH DENTAL PHOBIA

BY JOHN F. LHOTA, DMD

"I was never afraid of anything in the world –
except the dentist."

~ Taylor Caldwell, famous author

Many people equate the word "dentist" with "fear." Experts estimate that as many as seventy-five percent of adults in America experience some degree of dental fear, ranging from mild to severe. Five to ten percent of adults avoid the dentist at all costs, because they are so afraid of receiving dental treatment. They only go to the dentist when they have an extreme emergency, such as an agonizing toothache.

Such fear can sometimes make my chosen profession of dentistry a bit of a challenge—especially when the fear turns to anger. I still vividly remember the reaction of an eight year-old boy sitting in my dental chair after I informed him that he was going to need to have some work done.

He threatened to come back to my office and burn it down.

As far as I know, he was not related to the Soprano family, but when someone that age threatens you with arson, it tends to stay in your mind. I *am* comfortable, nevertheless, treating nervous patients; I *have* to be comfortable about this aspect of my work. After all, when the dentist is as anxious as the patient, the tension just doubles.

WHAT CAUSES DENTAL PHOBIA?

Dental phobia is a term used to describe a severe fear of the dentist, but I will be using it in this chapter to discuss that fear in general. I fortunately have never experienced it myself, and as a child, I was interested in teeth and liked my family dentist. When I was around thirteen, my childhood dentist even encouraged my interest in dentistry by inviting me to his office to watch him make a crown for my father.

Others *are not* so fortunate, and their fear of the dentist comes from one of two main causes: Direct Experience and Indirect Experience. Let's look at both of these individually.

- **Direct Experience**

Direct experience means you had a difficult, especially painful, or just plain unpleasant incident with a dentist. By the way, a painful procedure alone does not necessarily create this fear. The dentist's attitude may be a big, contributing factor towards development of dental phobia. One's ultimate impression of a dental visit may vary, depending on whether one perceives the dentist as warm, caring, and understanding, or cold, uninterested, and impersonal.

If you felt the dentist was honestly trying to help you to the fullest extent, you might not look back at the procedure negatively, even if it had been somewhat difficult. However, if the dentist had just plowed through the procedure, oblivious to your discomfort, this insensitivity and indifference might deter you from seeking future dental treatment.

Another direct experience that might cause avoidance of the dentist is the experience of unsatisfactory results from previous dental treatment. Perhaps the work was done several years ago, before recent improvements in technology. This type of experience can lead to loss of trust, even with different dental caregivers. Under these circumstances, a patient might only come in for basic check-ups and cleanings, but fail to address significant dental problems. Many patients may even fail to take care of obvious cosmetic concerns related to dental problems, and as a consequence, may feel socially awkward.

- **INDIRECT EXPERIENCE**

Indirect experience means your are afraid of the dentist due to outside influences, but not because of your own personal experiences in the dental office. This fear can develop in several ways:

  o **Vicarious Learning**

Vicarious learning is when other people in your life have conditioned you to be wary of the dentist. One patient of mine used to be teased by his older siblings, who exagger-

MORE THAN A MOUTHFUL

ated the size of the drill, telling him it was about five times as big as it actually was. Sometimes parents have their own strong anxiety about dental visits and communicate this anxiety to a child. Friends can also have traumatic experiences that they share, leaving a bad impression. How often do you hear about a friend's favorable dental visit?

- **Mass Media**

Anybody who has ever seen Steve Martin sing "Be a Dentist" while gleefully working on a screaming patient's mouth in the movie, "Little Shop of Horrors," knows that dentists are quick and easy punch lines for comedians, movies, and television shows.

I cannot tell you how many times, over the past twenty years, a patient has asked me, "Is it safe?" the question asked by the drill-wielding torturer in the old movie, "Marathon Man." Even though we strive to make our patients as comfortable as possible, the myth persists that a visit to the dentist is one of the most agonizing things that you can do in your life.

- **Other Stimulus**

Frequently, the fear of the dentist is actually transferred from other phobias; for example, a bad experience in another medical setting, such as a hospital or physician's office. Just the familiar smell of antiseptics can trigger a bad memory.

- **Lack of Control**

People who have been physically or emotionally abused may react negatively to feeling "helpless" in the dental chair, but even people who have not been abused in some way can experience much anxiety from feeling a lack of control during a dental appointment.

Such patients can often find comfort by sharing and explaining their feelings with their dentist The dentist and patient may agree on a patient's "stop" hand signal, to indicate a patient's need to pause during treatment, thus also giving the patient some control.

TREATING NERVOUS PATIENTS

When I'm faced with a nervous patient, the first thing I need to determine is the amount of fear the person has. Is this fear something that can be talked through or not? If not, then we often prescribe anti-anxiety medication before treatment.

For most people, this is not necessary. Empathy is the most important trait that dentists can bring to the table. By reassuring the patient that we will not hurt them and that we will treat them with compassion, we begin to create the necessary bond of trust that will allow the patient to feel comfortable about receiving dental care from us.

Sometimes it is important to put your money where your mouth is (pardon the pun). With one patient, we guaranteed that we would not charge him if we did anything to hurt him (I got this idea from a fellow dentist). Patients feel that you must be serious about making sure they have a good experience, if you are willing to risk your fee for their comfort.

The most important thing is to approach every patient as an individual. Every person is different and every person has different concerns and needs. Some people are just afraid of the noise of the drill---others do not like to have people putting their hands in their mouths. Some people want to endlessly talk about the treatment until they know every single aspect of it; others do not want any details at all. You learn to do what gives each patient the most peace of mind.

Although I am certainly willing to prescribe sedation medication to those who really require it, I find it more worthwhile to work with patients until they feel like they can do without it. A very small percentage of patients can only deal with dental treatment by being put to sleep, however, for most people who are "dental phobes," getting the dental work done and having it done well is usually what gets them past their anxiety. It is comparable to a fear of flying—for most people, once they have mustered up the courage to take a flight, and continue doing so over time, the fear begins to fade because of the familiarity. The more you do it, the better you feel about it—and for most people, it is as simple as that.

OVERCOMING THE FEAR

To illustrate that last point, I would like to relate the story of one patient of mine who has been with me for about 20 years. She is wonderful to treat now, but when I first started seeing her, it was very different. She would only come in every couple of years when she had a toothache or other big problem with her teeth, and she would see a different dentist every time. The reason? Well, she was very rude, short-tempered, and unpleasant with everyone in the office.

When she came in to the dental office with a broken tooth one day, it was my turn to see her. She needed a root canal first and was very unhappy about it. I suggested, apparently for the first time, that she try some sedation medication—valium in this case—so she could deal with the procedure more positively. She agreed.

That one suggestion opened up many doors: whereas before

she only came in to handle specific problems as quickly as possible, now she started to return for subsequent visits to complete treatment. After that, she became a regular dental patient of mine for over two decades.

As the years have passed, she has needed less ad less medication to get through a treatment—and has become much more pleasant. Because I took the time to address her anxiety, she began to trust me, a trust that has been built over time.

If you have a dentist who is sensitive to your needs and is willing to work with a patient with dental phobia, you will probably find a way to deal with your ongoing dental treatment in a comfortable and relaxing way. A dentist who is insensitive to a patient's anxiety, however, can set you back a long way.

That is why it really comes down to selecting the right dentist. You want to make sure that the dentist does not mind taking the time to work with someone who is nervous. But if you feel like the dentist does not really care—or if the dentist is as nervous as you are about the prospect of your treatment-- then you are in the wrong office.

MAXIMIZING YOUR MINDSET

Yes, selecting the right dentist is very important—but is also helps if patients do some work on their own to help themselves work through their anxiety. I would like to end this chapter with a few tips on how to maximize your frame of mind and approach the dentist with the best possible attitude:

- *Remember that your fears are normal*

Do you recall that statistic that I quoted at the start of this chapter? I'll repeat it here—seventy –five percent of adults are fearful to some degree of dental treatments. Most keep it under control and consult with caring dentists who will put them at ease. The other important thing to realize is that dentists have more training in dealing with fearful patients now and have many tools and techniques available to minimize a patient's discomfort. Do not be embarrassed about coming in to see the dentist and first just talking honestly about your anxiety.

- ***Remember that sedation is an option***

Nitrous oxide, local anesthetics, and a sedative pill before your appointment are all different ways of assuring that your pain will be either minimal or non-existent. It is always important to take the first step toward dental health, even if you are one of the few patients who might require sleep sedation.

- ***Remember that you do not have to do it all at once***

If you wish, you can make your first visit just a consult—a chat with the dentist to make sure that you are comfortable with him or her. The next appointment could be a general examination, and the next might be the actual start of treatment. The right dentist will explain all the steps to you and make sure you know exactly what will happen during every visit (that is, if you want to know!)

- **Remember that you can control your environment**

It might help if you bring in your own music. Many dentists are also set up to allow you to watch DVD's . You might even bring along a family member or friend for moral support. Discuss with your dentist the different ways you can achieve a higher comfort level in the treatment room.

- **Remember to think positively**

If you dwell on horrible things that could but almost certainly will not, happen in the dental chair, you will only stoke the fires of your own fear. Remember that the people at a dental office are dedicated professionals who want you to have the best possible care – they are not your enemy. Work with them closely as you can, and you are bound to see favorable results!

If you experience dental phobia, then the two main points that I would like you to take away from this chapter are: (1) you need to be able to discuss your fear, and (2) you need to find the right dentist. A dentist who is able to meet you halfway when it comes to your anxiety will also be able to help you reach your goals of good dental health and a fabulous smile.

ABOUT JOHN

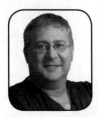

Dr. John Lhota is a 1985 graduate of the University of Pennsylvania School of Dental Medicine. He attended a six-year accelerated program for dentistry in conjunction with Rensselaer Polytechnic Institute for academically gifted students, which enabled him to obtain both his B.S. in Biology (minor in Literature) and his D.M.D. dental degree within a span of six years. He also holds a faculty appointment at the New York University College of Dentistry.

Dr. Lhota has been a practicing dentist in New York City for 25 years, providing comprehensive dental care with an emphasis on conservative quality care. Dr. Lhota is a distinguished member of the ADA, NY County Dental Society, Academy of General Dentistry, Crown Council, Sierra Club, and a supporter of the North Shore Animal League.

He lives in Manhattan with his wife, son, and two dogs, Yogurt and Dancer, both pugs. He is an animal lover and is fond of music.

CHAPTER 14

FIVE LIFE RISKS YOUR DENTIST CAN HELP YOU AVOID

BY SCOTT SCHUMANN, DDS

"The part can never be well unless the whole is well."

~ Plato

'll admit that the title of this chapter was meant to grab you; however, it's also very, very TRUE. What happens in your mouth affects your overall health to a greater degree than any medical professional ever thought possible. It's only been in the last 10 to 20 years that we've discovered just how important good oral health is to the rest of your body – and the huge impact it can have when it comes to heart disease, cancer, diabetes and other maladies.

You might say that your dental health is a lot like the engine in a car. If you don't take care of that engine and give it regular tune-ups, eventually the car will stop working. It's the same thing with how well you take care of your teeth and gums – neglect your oral care and it will eventually impact vital systems in your body. And that means illness, disease and other unpleasant outcomes.

Even looking past overall health issues, neglecting your teeth can also lead to a tremendous psychological problem – low self-esteem. "Avoiders" who stay away from the dentist often end up with broken and discolored teeth, as well as a strong bad breath problem – this causes a lot of problems in their interactions with others. When someone who hasn't been to the dentist in years and years finally comes in to our practice and goes through our suggested treatment, the difference in their personality before and after is often like night and day. They're happier, less guarded, friendlier – and willing to show their teeth when they smile.

In this chapter, I'd like to explore in a little more depth the importance of what's called the oral-systemic connection – the crucial link between the health of your mouth and your overall wellness – by examining five serious issues that can be created by dental neglect.

RISK #1:
HEART DISEASE

For most of you, this will be a big shocker: The American Heart Association's research shows that poor oral health could increase your chances of developing heart disease - *even more so than high cholesterol and triglyceride levels.*

The source of the danger to your heart? Periodontal infections – or, in other words, gum disease. Gum disease is caused by plaque buildup and affects around 75% of American adults – and almost 30% show signs of the more severe disease, chronic periodontitis. This is particularly alarming because, as you'll see as you continue on with this chapter, gum disease is the culprit in almost every serious health issue that bad oral health can trigger.

Your next question probably is – how does what happens to my gums affect other organs in my body? Well, a lot of bacteria is involved with periodontal infections – and it can easily enter your bloodstream, attach to blood vessel and increase clot formations. As many of you already know, clots decrease the blood supply flow to the heart and can increase your chances of a heart attack.

One study done in the U.S., which looked at the data for almost 10,000 people, showed that those with periodontitis had a 25% increased risk of coronary heart disease compared to those with little or no periodontal disease. For men under 50, periodontal disease was an even bigger risk factor – they had nearly *twice* the risk of coronary heart disease compared to men who had little or no gum disease.

RISK #2:
THE DANGER OF DIABETES

Gum disease can actually induce diabetes as well. Again, bacteria from your mouth can enter your bloodstream; but, in addition to causing clots, it can also activate your immune cells.

These activated cells produce inflammatory biological

signals called "cytokines" that can have a very harsh effect throughout your entire body. And when it comes to diabetes, the cells in your pancreas that are responsible for insulin production can be damaged or even destroyed by chronic high levels of cytokines. And that's where Type 2 diabetes can happen — even in otherwise healthy individuals with no other risk factors for diabetes.

If you are already diabetic, good oral care becomes critical. The problems controlling blood sugar caused by both Type 1 and Type 2 diabetes affect the mouth in various ways, including:

- **Dry Mouth** – Increased blood sugar can lead to a decrease in saliva, causing dry mouth.
- **Gingivitis and Periodontal Disease** – Diabetes reduces the body's ability to fight infections, so it's easier for the bacteria normally present in the mouth to overwhelm those defenses and for gum disease to take hold.
- **Slow Healing** – Diabetes reduces blood flow, so it's more difficult for the mouth to heal after oral surgery.
- **Thrush** – The high levels of sugar found in diabetic saliva – along with decreased resistance – can lead to this fungal infection in the mouth.

For these reasons and more, it's especially important for diabetics to see their dentists regularly. A dentist will often work with a diabetic patient's medical doctor to come up with a care plan that works for them. This means knowing what medications the patient is currently taking, being aware of the patient's blood sugar levels during treatments, and taking their condition into account when scheduling any oral surgery or other serious procedures.

FIVE LIFE RISKS YOUR DENTIST CAN HELP YOU AVOID

In addition, the dentist and his or her staff should work with his or her diabetic patients to keep their mouths free of harmful bacteria, monitor their dental health and tackle any infections promptly, before they get out of control. This helps protect the patient's teeth – which are also incredibly important to diabetics.

Here's why: a new study done in Australia, conducted by The George Institute for International Health in Sydney, Australia, discovered that diabetics who lose all of their teeth are twice as likely to die as diabetics in the same age group who have managed to keep the majority of their teeth.

The study covered almost 11,000 adults who were aged 55 to 88, all of them with Type 2 diabetes. And the results are, frankly, frightening. During the five years the study monitored them, twice as many diabetics without teeth died.

This is especially disturbing because diabetic patients are naturally prone to gum disease, and gum disease is the number one cause of tooth loss. The bottom line is that if you're diabetic and putting off visiting the dentist for any reason, it's probably time to pick up the phone and schedule a check-up now. If you've already lost teeth, dental implants may be able to protect your remaining natural teeth by keeping the bone around them healthy and alive.

RISK #3:
THE CANCER THREAT

Periodontal infections put men at an elevated risk of not only heart disease, but also cancer. Research published recently in *The Lancet Oncology*, a leading general medical journal, found that men with a history of gum disease are

14 percent more likely to develop cancer than men with healthy gums. In fact, researchers uncovered that men with periodontal disease may be 49 percent more likely to develop kidney cancer and 30 percent more likely to develop blood cancers.

Another recent study by the Dana-Farber Cancer Institute and the Harvard School of Public Health establishes a pretty strong link between periodontal disease and pancreatic cancer. The study, eliminating all risk factors for pancreatic cancer (such as age, body mass index, smoking, etc.), discovered that those with gum disease were *63% more likely* to develop pancreatic cancer than those who didn't have periodontal disease.

What's the scientific explanation of this? Again, it comes to bacteria from the mouth getting into the bloodstream and causing inflammation. This inflammation could theoretically promote the growth of cancer cells, but this is an area that is still being researched.

RISK #4
CHRONIC BAD BREATH

Okay, it may not be as serious as heart disease or cancer, but bad breath can certainly make your life miserable in a myriad of other ways, as hundreds of TV commercials over the years have shown us. Whether at home with family, at the office or in the midst of any social interaction, bad breath, officially known as halitosis, can lead to constant embarrassment and avoidance of any close contact with others.

Bad breath is caused by bacteria which break down proteins already in the mouth. These proteins, and other materials which are in the mouth either naturally or from what we eat and drink, are the real power behind bad breath.

There are three major areas where halitosis can happen:

- **The Tongue**

The tongue is a popular place for the development of bad breath in mouths that are healthy or are infected with gum disease. It could be caused by the amount of bacterial coating on the tongue, and/or the presences of deep fissures or grooves on the tongue. Cleaning your tongue is important to battling bad breath – there can be up to one hundred times the amount of bacteria on it than there would be if you brushed it clean.

- **The Teeth**

Teeth can also be covered with the bacteria that cause bad breath (and if they are, keep in mind that you can probably assume the tongue is overloaded with the stuff too). The biggest areas of concern would be the sides of teeth that touch one another, because you can't get at them with a toothbrush and must use floss to clean them.

- **The Gums**

Gum tissues are another prime suspect for bad breath. They can form a "sulcus," which is basically a ditch that goes around the tooth and is usually 1-3 millimeters in depth. If you have gum disease, this ditch deepens and is called a "pocket." Bacteria can get into these pockets and easily cause bad breath.

By the way, if you continue to have bad breath after you've cleaned your tongue as well as brushed and floss, your body is most likely trying to alert you to the fact that you have gum disease. And considering everything you've learned so far about what gum disease can do to the rest of your body, you should definitely visit your friendly neighborhood dentist to take care of it.

RISK #5:
LOSING YOUR SMILE

In terms of appearance, the biggest danger that results from avoiding the dentist is losing your teeth. Some people still regard tooth loss as they age as an inevitability, so they might not do everything they can to keep their teeth – and their smile – into their golden years.

Well, the fact is that tooth loss *can* be prevented over the long haul of life – but not without regular brushing, flossing and dental check-ups. Once gum disease rears its ugly head and is left unchecked, you end up with swelling, bleeding, pain and redness of gums…which leads eventually to the loss of teeth.

If you've got a winning smile, there's no reason you can't keep it. And if you're not happy with your smile as is, there's no reason that today's cosmetic dentistry technology can't make it more to your liking.

FOR A LONGER HEALTHIER LIFE, PRACTICE GOOD DENTAL HEALTH HABITS

As I've mentioned in this chapter, the science on the links between gum disease and other illnesses is still relatively new. The links have definitely been established, but more research is needed to understand the how and why of them.

The important takeaway from all this, however, is that the links *are* real – and it's more crucial than ever before to practice good dental health habits. You can also avail yourself of several additional home products – rinses and other special tools – that can help keep your mouth healthier in between office visits. We are currently planning to offer the best of these for sale in our own offices.

I'm proud to help my patients attain better health in all areas through my practice. I hope you permit your dentist to do the same for you. Dentistry isn't just about filling cavities anymore – it's about looking good, feeling good and living a long, healthy and active life. And I hope that's just what your experience will be throughout your lifetime.

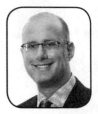

ABOUT SCOTT

Dr Scott Schumann graduated from the Ohio State University Dental School in 1989 and then completed his residency training at the University of Texas Health Science Center at San Antonio in 1991, a phenomenal experience, being trained and certified in advanced dental techniques, dental implants, and sedation dentistry. He also received a fellowship in Hospital Dentistry, helping him to excel in assisting his medically compromised patients. After returning to Columbus Ohio, Dr. Schumann started his career and began teaching in the Advanced Dentistry Clinic at the Ohio State University, teaching dental residents advanced cosmetic, implant, hospital, and sedation dentistry for ten years.

Dr Schumann's office in Grove City, a suburb 8 minutes south of downtown Columbus, Ohio, is often referred to by clients as "fun" and "cool." Dr. Schumann and his staff recently won "Best Team in the Nation" honors out of 1200 dental offices, and are well known for their love of helping their patients achieve the smile they always dreamed of. His highly trained professional team and office, with amazing new technological advancements, makes each patient visit as fun as possible without guilt or embarrassment.

Scott is an active member in the Columbus Dental Society, Ohio Dental Association, American Dental Association, Academy of General Dentists, American Academy of Cosmetic Dentists, Dental Organization for Conscious Sedation, and the American Dental Society of Anesthesiology has been very beneficial in keeping him and his team up to date on the latest developments in dentistry.

Dr Scott Schumann, a Best-Selling Author, has been published in multiple research journals, featured in chapters in *Oral-Facial Emergencies*, The 21 Principles of Smile Design, and the #1 best selling books *Shift Happens*, *Power Principles of Success*, *ROI Marketing Secrets*, and *Game Changers – The World's Leading Entrepreneurs*. The forthcoming book that he has co-authored, *More Than A Mouthful*, will feature top advice from some of the most successful dental professionals from across the country. The authors will be discussing how total body health starts in the mouth.

Dr. Scott has been quoted in the **USA Today, The Wall St. Journal, Newsweek** and appeared in the Fall of 2009 on America's PremierExperts® TV show on NBC, CBS, ABC and FOX and interviewed on the radio show the Next Big Thing®. Dr Scott Schumann's company, Grove City Dental, was recently recognized on **Inc. 5000** 2010 and 2011 Lists for America's Fastest-Growing Private Companies.

Dr Scott Schumann a native of Columbus, Ohio, grew up loving the Buckeyes, playing sports, and collecting rocks. Dr Schumann and his wife Robin live in downtown Columbus with their dog Bourbon, the boxer. Dr Schumann loves supporting the local arts, sponsoring little league teams, golfing, fishing, attending concerts and NASCAR events.

For more information, please visit:

http://www.AmericasPremierDentist.com
http://www.SnoozeThroughItDentisty.com
http://www.GoodHealthStartsInYourMouth.com

CHAPTER 15

TREATING PERIODONTITIS

BY STEVE JOHNSON, DDS

(PERIOLASE - This chapter is about a new alternative for the treatment of moderate to severe periodontal disease that has FDA approval via the use of the Periolase and LANAP procedure. In order to discuss the Periolase and the LANAP procedure, a basic understanding of what periodontal disease is, its effects, and how it can be treated follows.)

Periodontal disease is a progressive disorder that affects the soft tissue and bone which supports the teeth. It is a disease that three out of four people will have to some degree in their lifetime. In the United States, over 100 million people have moderate to severe periodontal disease and less than five percent are getting treatment yearly. These numbers do not include those with the early stages of the disease. Many people, because the tissue is inflamed, keeping the tissue at a normal level around the base of the tooth, never realize there is a problem until they notice that a tooth has become slightly loose. In this respect, periodontal disease is insidious, giving people a false sense of security that all is well. Unfortunately, this keeps people out of the dental office until very late in the disease progression.

The early stage of the disease is called gingivitis. It is the inflammation of the gums around the teeth. Gingivitis occurs in response to the buildup of plaque, tartar (calculus) and its associated bacteria on the teeth. Gingivitis is the body's immune response to these bacteria and their byproducts. A consequence of this is bleeding gums. Ironically, at this stage, a dental cleaning, daily flossing and brushing can prevent any further advancement of the disease process. The damage from gingivitis may be reversed once the teeth have been professionally cleaned and home care instructions are followed. However, it takes ten to fourteen days for the gum bleeding to stop and the tissue to return to a healthy state.

Over time, if the gingivitis is not treated and resolved, bacteria will infiltrate into the gingival tissue surrounding the teeth, and as a result, the body's immune response will become more involved. As the body fights this bacterial invasion, bone support of the teeth will be lost. Deep gum pockets are created next to the teeth as the gingival attachment to the teeth starts to break down. Eventually, the teeth become loose and perhaps this is the stage where people first notice that they have a problem. They may have also had someone tell them that they have bad breath. All this breakdown of support structures around the teeth, with the inflammatory response to the bacteria and its byproducts, allows the bacteria a route of entry into the circulatory system through the vascular network which surrounds our teeth.

The invasion of bacteria into our circulatory system has been linked to multiple systemic disorders. Plaque build-up in our arteries is generally known to be related to high cholesterol but may also be due to the bacterial onslaught from periodontal disease and an immune response in the bloodstream – where the body tries to capture and elimi-nate bacteria in the bloodstream. Heart attacks and strokes can be caused by bacterial plaques that have dislodged and traveled to the heart and brain. The possibility of deleteri-ous effects on other organs of the body cannot be ruled out.

There is some evidence to suggest that there is a link be-tween periodontal disease and preterm birth. Preterm birth (less than 37 weeks gestation) is the leading cause of neo-natal mortality in the United States affecting 11% of all live births. Data suggests that a chronic oral infection like peri-odontal disease may contribute to preeclampsia, preterm birth, fetal growth restriction, and fetal loss.

In periodontitis, oral gram-negative anaerobic bacteria (those which require no oxygen for survival) predominate. The methods by which they destroy tissue are both direct from bacterial byproducts and indirect through bacterial in-fection and the body's inflammatory and immune responses. Some risk factors for development of periodontal disease are advancing age, diabetes and smoking. It is known there is a risk factor for atherosclerosis and rheumatoid arthritis. Periodontitis is common in women of child-bearing years.

From the time we start to eat food as infants, bacteria has played a role in digestion. Without bacteria, we would not be able to break the food down and obtain the very nutrients needed for our survival. We have a mutually beneficial relationship that serves both the bacteria and ourselves. This relationship for digestion is supposed to be a closed system. What this means is that the bacteria present in the mouth and gut have no direct access to the circulatory system. The lining of epithelium and mucosa is to act as a barrier to any and all invaders (bacteria) to the rest of the body. With periodontal disease and the associated bleeding gums, bacteria are given the means to enter the bloodstream directly. In a healthy state, this does not happen.

Dentistry has made many strides over the last 100 years. The application of scientific research and clinical studies from the 1950's forward have led to better treatment modalities and even prevention of many of the ailments that lead to early tooth loss. Fluoride in drinking water, fluoride in toothpaste has decreased dental decay. Development of the high-speed handpiece made dental work more comfortable. Root canals have given one the ability to retain an internally dead tooth. However, it took physicians the first half of the last century to accept them as a valid treatment for an abscessed tooth. Dental implants were developed and gave one the means to replace lost teeth without the need for a partial or full denture.

Dentistry has progressed from its roots as a more technical field of dealing with the consequences of dental problems, i.e., abscesses, lost teeth, broken teeth, and thus a reactive model of treatment, to more proactive model, treating the underlying disease process with emphasis on prevention. The treatment of periodontal disease is a prime example of this.

Dentists in the eras prior to the 1960's primarily placed fillings, crowns, bridges, extracted teeth, and placed partials or dentures. Teeth were cleaned but periodontal disease was not understood. Research in the 1960's and 1970's led to a better understanding of periodontal disease. It was found that like many other chronic diseases, the disease could be managed. The management of periodontal disease involved doing whatever was necessary to remove tartar and bacteria from the teeth both above the gum and below. This varied with the progression of the disease and in the more advanced forms, was much more invasive. Another component to treatment involved teaching the patient better home care techniques for brushing and flossing. The 'water pik' came into vogue around this time as an augmentation to home-care techniques.

The research found that once a person was treated for their periodontal condition, more frequent dental maintenance would be necessary due to the length of time it would take for a mature bacterial colony to form in the sulcular pocket surrounding the treated teeth. It was found that a mature colony of bad bacteria would take only 90 to 120 days to form. From this data, return visits for dental cleanings were set on a three or four month basis. If a patient could be maintained without further bone loss at four months, they kept on a four month recall schedule. If on the other hand, this did not maintain stability of their periodontal disease, a three-month recall was set.

Periodontal treatment was all about pocket elimination. In a state of good health, the depth of the sulcus around a tooth is 1 to 3mm. In an unhealthy state, the readings are much beyond that. Research found in the deeper areas beyond 3mm, as the depth increased, the amount of anaerobic gram-negative bacteria increased.

Traditional treatment of periodontal disease varies according to the severity of the person's condition. When there are few pockets ranging from 4-6mm in depth, the only necessary treatment may be scaling and root planing followed by more frequent recall. Scaling and root planing is the process by which the tartar and bacteria are mechanically removed from the surface of the tooth and root in the periodontal pocket around the tooth. If there is diseased or inflamed tissue, some of this is removed during the process. This procedure is done while the area is numbed via local anesthesia. This is done with both hand instruments and ultrasonic scalers, some of which use antibacterial solutions as their lubricant.

When the periodontal disease is moderate to severe with pockets deeper than 6mm, traditionally a periodontist would surgically expose the area under anesthesia to visibly see the defects in the bone and visibly see where the tartar is that must be removed. After the procedure, it may become necessary to attach the gum tissue back to the teeth by suturing at a much higher level on the root than prior to surgery. This surgically reduces the pocket depth to a normal 1 to 3mm, making the pockets easier to maintain with home care and helps eliminate the environment that tended to harbor the anaerobic bacteria colonies creating the immune/host inflammation response leading to the bone loss. The downside to this type of surgery was the appearance of long teeth due to root exposure from surgery. Some people ended up with root sensitivity from this additional exposure of tooth structure – which under normal circumstances was covered with gum tissue. This was a necessary trade off in order to regain gingival health and to be able to manage the periodontal disease. The upside for the patient is that the teeth were not lost. The downside was, in some cases, teeth that looked <u>long</u>. Increased temperature sensitivity and a greater amount of exposed tooth structure that had to be kept clean.

From my clinical experience of patients I have seen over the past 20 years, those that have had traditional periodontal surgery have kept their teeth, but the issue has been maintaining these longer teeth (exposed roots). Generally, all patients have had problems with cleaning them. Invariably, the exposed roots which are organic structures, versus inorganic like enamel, become prone to dental decay. The roots just are not as resistant to decay and they are not as easily repaired when decay occurs. Composite fillings were developed to <u>bond</u> to enamel; they do not <u>bond</u> as strongly to an organic structure. Additionally, as we age, we may become more prone to decay due to changes in our saliva and the natural antibodies secreted in it.

Another cause of the increased root decay is the increased number of medications that a person may be taking. A large percentage of medications can cause a drying effect on the mouth via a decrease in saliva. Blood pressure medications, depression medications, and sinus medications are all example of medications that can add to a dry oral environment.

The options in the treatment of periodontal disease have remained somewhat the same over the past couple of decades. When problems have been severe and teeth have been lost, advancement in the areas of dental implants has given new hope to those who have lost some of their teeth. The incidence of surgery, cutting the gum, and suturing have remained the same. Attempts have been made to regain lost bone, and when pockets are isolated interproximally between the teeth with a wall of bone to the sides, there can be some gain of lost bone. There are also ways to surgically augment recessed gingiva to some degree. There has been some success with this <u>as well.</u>

An alternative approach for treatment of moderate to severe periodontal disease was developed by Drs. Robert H. Gregg II, DDS and Delvin K. McCarthy, DDS. Both have been pioneers in the use of <u>Nd:YAG</u> lasers in treating periodontal disease. They co-founded Millennium Dental Technologies, Inc. and co-developed the FDA cleared Periolase pulsed <u>Nd:YAG</u> laser. They co-developed the patented laser ENAP periodontal technique (LANAP).

LANAP (Laser Assisted New Attachment Procedure) or LPT (Laser Periodontal Therapy) is a technique developed to treat periodontal disease without surgically cutting the gums, laying flap and sewing (stitching) it back. It is accomplished by first removing the tartar from the teeth with small instruments and ultrasonics. Once this is done, the Millennium Periolase's small glass fiber is placed between the gums and the tooth where controlled measured light energy is applied. This energy is in such a wavelength that it affects some of the diseased gum tissue and the bacteria present in the pockets around the teeth. The area is then cleansed and the fiber is placed once again in the pocket to aid in the formation of a fibrous clot around the tooth. There is no cutting, flapping or suturing of the gums. The gum tissue does not recede like with periodontal surgery. The fibrous clot aids in the body's healing potential.

Patients must follow a strict protocol to maximize the healing potential of the body. In surgery there is a forced compliance of the patient. In LANAP, compliance is voluntary; the patient's compliance to guidelines in home care will affect the degree of <u>possible</u> regeneration of bone and attachment to the teeth. In addition, the occlusion has to be adjusted so that no excessive force is applied to any one tooth. Teeth that have mobility must be splinted (bonded to other teeth) to stabilize them so that regeneration is maximized.

As with other forms of periodontal treatment, a three-month recall is necessary. The teeth will not be probed to check healing for at least nine months so that the development of new attachment is not disturbed.

LANAP/LPT must be performed by a dental professional that is trained in the practice and use of the Periolase through the Institute For Advanced Laser Dentistry. The Periolase and LANAP/LPT is <u>not</u> a cure for periodontal disease; however, it may reverse some of the damage caused by the disease. There is a potential for a gain in attachment and possibly bone regeneration. It has the additional advantage of requiring no cutting or flapping for suturing, thereby greatly reducing the possibility of post-operative pain.

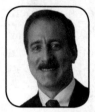

ABOUT STEVEN

Dr. Steven Johnson leads a highly successful dental practice in Northern Virginia. His practice grosses in the top one percent of the country. As a comprehensive restorative dentist for over 25 years, Steve's focus is to provide excellent oral health care to his patients. With dedication and commitment, he leads his professional team members, by example, to strive for excellence and compassion in the field of dentistry. Steve resides in Springfield, Virginia with his lovely wife, Penny and their son, Andrew.

CHAPTER 16

IT'S NEVER TOO LATE

BY CHRIS PORT, DMD

"It is never too late to be what you might have been."
~ George Eliot

t's never too late. That's what people say when it comes to love and romance, travel and adventure, going back to school and improving yourself...even to what you do for a living at the moment. It's certainly not, however, a phrase you instantly associate with the dentist - but the fact of the matter is that it *is* never too late to have the smile you've always dreamed of having.

Especially today, the science of technology and the art of cosmetic dentistry have progressed to the point where, in the vast majority of cases, we can completely transform the look of anyone's teeth – no matter how they've been neglected or ignored over the years.

I know from first-hand experience that in many cases, the people who stop going to the dentist for an extended period of time – a year or so – begin to worry about what's going on in their mouth. Unfortunately, that anxiety frequently doesn't cause them to come right back to the dentist to check it out – instead, it makes them afraid to find out what's going on. So they continue to ignore the situation, continue to postpone going to the dentist and continue to allow their oral health to degenerate.

No matter how long you've put off going to the dentist, though, you can still turn things around. Obviously, the faster you take action, the less treatment you'll need; it may just be a matter of a good cleaning, polishing and whitening to transform a dull and dingy smile to a bright and beautiful one. But if your dental problems have grown to be much more than that, a trustworthy and skilled dentist will take your nerves into account and put you at as much ease as possible in order to do what it takes to help you regain your smile and health.

I'd like to share one special patient story in this chapter that illustrates exactly how making the decision to finally trust a dentist can literally change someone's life. But first I'd like to talk about how a dentist changed my life.

THE UNDERGROUND DENTIST

Yes, I can safely say that a dentist certainly made a huge difference to me. That dentist just happened to be my grandfather.

And that makes me feel lucky. Most people grow up being scared of the dentist – either they had bad experiences as children or because their parents *made* it into a bad experience (there are moms and dads who actually threaten their misbehaving kids with a trip to the dentist – wonderful news for us who have to later face those kids!).

I grew up with a totally different perspective because of my grandfather. By this time, he had officially retired from dentistry – but he had so many patients that wanted to continue to see him, he actually put a small dental office in his basement! He had a little waiting area, a little room for lab work, and another room for examining patients which, yes, contained the traditional dental patient chair – all there in the cellar.

A lot of kids played with train sets, pool tables and other games in their grandparents' basement. Well, my brother and I would hang out and play with our toys in my grandfather's dental office – and naturally, I gained an interest in what dentistry was all about. Because I knew I was good with my hands – I built small model cars and trains as a boy – I figured I would be good at it. And fortunately, I was smart enough to learn everything I needed to know at the Medical College of Georgia, based in Augusta.

That education, by the way, hasn't stopped as I've continued in my dental career. In the last 8 or 9 years of my 13 years practicing dentistry, I've had the opportunity to work with several world-renowned leaders in cosmetic dentistry, enabling me to learn techniques from the top people in my field. This has aided me in providing the latest, cutting-edge treatments to my patients.

And it's also why I can confidently say it is never too late to save your smile. I know the miracles that can be easily accomplished with today's technology.

THIRTY YEARS WITHOUT A SMILE

One such "miracle" was one of the most memorable patient treatments I've ever undertaken. When people avoid the dentist for twenty or thirty years, they just don't understand the choices they now have in terms of fixing their smile. They're afraid to do anything because they have no idea what can be done, because they've been "out of the loop" for so long.

One man I ended up treating was definitely in this category. He literally had not had any serious dental treatment in 30 years. When he was young, he had a few serious dental injuries due to the sports he played. At the time, he had some dental work done to try and repair the damage – but, he told me, the treatment was always painful and, whenever they finished, the work didn't look very good. These experiences convinced him that going to a dentist was just opening himself up to agonizing appointments that wouldn't bring the results he wanted them to have.

Finally, his attitude, hardened in his late teens, became, "Why should I let these people put me through all that discomfort, why should I put in all that time and effort…if my teeth are still going to look bad?" So he put his smile away for three decades and stayed away from the dentist, except for minimal check-ups, because he didn't think anything could really be done about his appearance and he was angry about what he had gone through. He had lost trust in dentistry's ability to really fix anything.

His problem, however, was that his job as a golf pro forced him, more and more, to interact with the public – and not just the average everyday public, but the high-end clientele that frequented the private golf course where he worked.

Meanwhile, the condition of his teeth grew worse and worse, to the point where teeth began to break off.

He still wouldn't submit to any dental treatment that might address his unsightly smile - but he grew more and more embarrassed by his appearance. He even grew a full beard and moustache to distract anyone from looking at his mouth. Whenever there was a camera in sight, he tried to duck out of the photos, and, whenever he couldn't manage that, he wore a painful grimace instead of a genuine smile when the picture was snapped.

Finally, he began to get weary of hiding his teeth and his smile. He was sick of feeling bad about the way he looked, he wasn't getting any younger and he wanted to be more social and start dating. He made the decision to explore his options to see if he could turn things around.

That's when he came to see us, hoping dentistry nowadays was different than it had been when he was a teenager; it had been so long since he had sought treatment, he truly had no idea what could be done. We sat down with him, went over his X-rays, talked about what was possible and, most importantly to him, we listened to his history and his concerns. The main theme of what he was saying was, "If I'm going to do something about this, I don't want to go through all the treatment and still be unhappy after all the time and expense."

We reassured him and began the treatment. We started with his gum issues and did nonsurgical gum therapy to get them healthy again. Then we did some cosmetic dentistry to rebuild the pieces of his teeth that were broken down. Despite all his qualms and reservations, he went through the process without a complaint and acted as if he was comfortable with everything we were doing. We were able to complete everything without a hitch – and, best of all, his new smile looked terrific.

A few months ago, he came in for a follow-up visit, to make sure everything was working out all right for him. And the coolest thing about it is that he did something that I've never had any other patient do in my 13 years as a practicing dentist.

He was all excited and ran up to me, saying, "You've got to see this!" Then he pulled out his wallet and yanked out his driver's license. He said, "Here, look at this – I just got this new license two weeks ago."

I took a look at it – and my eyes went to the photo of him on the license, in which he was sporting a huge toothy grin. I looked back up at him – and he was beaming with pride.

"I have not smiled for a driver's license photo since I was 16," he told me. Every time he had renewed his license, he never cracked a grin – and he was now 50 years old.

For someone to be that excited about something as small as a driver's license photo was truly phenomenal. And it indicated a giant change overall in his personality had oc- curred. When we first met him, he was in a little bit of a shell, not difficult or nasty, just very restrained and re- served. Now, since he had his smile restored, he was trans- formed, both in how he interacted with others and how he felt about himself. The only word I can think of to fully describe this change is "rejuvenated."

DON'T BE AFRAID TO TAKE ACTION

By the way, it's not just us "mere mortals" who can sometimes put off the dentist too long – even the rich and famous share in this unhealthy procrastination. Whoopi Goldberg, movie and TV star and current host of "The View" on ABC, had her own brush with dental disaster. And she made an important point on the program about how it's not just about appearance – your very life could be at stake.

Like many people, the actress and comedienne neglected her dental care – to the point where she wound up with a serious periodontal infection that will lead to the loss of some of her teeth and, left unchecked, might have damaged her overall health and even threatened her life. On "The View," Goldberg pointed out a fact that dentists have known for years – that there is a strong connection between dental health and overall health.

Gum disease, in particular, can affect the health of your heart, your pancreas and can elevate your chances of having a stroke. It can even bring on diabetes or aggravate the condition of a diabetic.

So, if you have been putting off that visit to the dentist for too long, pick up the phone and make that appointment. As with anything else, the sooner you take action, the easier it will be to address any problems – and the healthier and happier a life you will have.

I'm very serious about the happiness element too. As I tell my staff, our patients aren't buying procedures – they're buying how they feel *about* themselves after the procedures. When people get their smiles back, it helps them restore their confidence in themselves and interact comfortably in social situations.

It's never too late to get back that smile and ensure your overall health. However – and here is where I will contradict myself a little bit – it *can* be too late if you allow your oral health to worsen to the point where major things go wrong.

For example, losing your permanent teeth is never a desirable outcome. Although we can do incredible things with dental implants to solve the problem of missing teeth, the best scenario for all of us is to keep as many of our natural teeth as possible as long as possible. Also, as just noted, permanent health issues can flare up as a result of serious gum disease – issues that aren't easily disposed of, if they can be disposed of at all.

The answer to all of the above is simple; schedule regular dentist appointments and keep them. Your oral health is important to your appearance, your health, your social life and your overall well-being.

Yes, it's never too late to fix your smile...but it's always better not to be late at all.

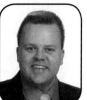

ABOUT CHRIS

Dr. Forest Christopher Port is a full-time practicing dentist in Asheville, North Carolina.

In 2007, Dr. Port founded the Asheville Smile Center, a dental practice dedicated to helping patients achieve a lifetime of dental health and beautiful smiles. Utilizing advanced materials and equipment, and implementing innovative techniques, the team at the Asheville Smile Center help to restore the lost confidence (suffered by millions of adults) of their patients – due to worn out, broken-down, crooked and discolored teeth and smiles.

In addition to his practice, Dr. Port spends time with his wife Heather and his two wonderful children, Hailey and Hunter, enjoying the beautiful mountains of Western North Carolina.

For more information about Dr. Chris Port and the Asheville Smile Center, please visit: www.AshevilleSmileCenter.com.